Creative Engagement

A Johns Hopkins Press Health Book

Creative Engagement

A HANDBOOK OF ACTIVITIES FOR PEOPLE WITH DEMENTIA

Rachael Wonderlin

With Geri M. Lotze, PhD

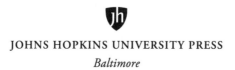

JOHNS HOPKINS UNIVERSITY PRESS

Baltimore

Note to the Reader: This book is not meant to substitute for medical care, and treatment should not be based solely on its contents. Instead, treatment must be developed in a dialogue between the individual and his or her physician. This book has been written to help with that dialogue.

© 2020 Johns Hopkins University Press
All rights reserved. Published 2020
Printed in the United States of America on acid-free paper
9 8 7 6 5 4 3 2 1

Johns Hopkins University Press
2715 North Charles Street
Baltimore, Maryland 21218-4363
www.press.jhu.edu

Library of Congress Cataloging-in-Publication Data

Names: Wonderlin, Rachael, 1989– author.
Title: Creative engagement : a handbook of activities for people with dementia /
    Rachael Wonderlin. With Geri M. Lotze, PhD.
Description: Baltimore : Johns Hopkins University Press, 2020. | Series: A Johns Hopkins
    Press health book | Includes bibliographical references and index.
Identifiers: LCCN 2019023261 | ISBN 9781421437279 (hardcover) | ISBN
    9781421437286 (paperback) | ISBN 9781421437293 (ebook)
Subjects: LCSH: Dementia—Patients—Care. | Dementia—Patients—Recreation. |
    Dementia—Patients—Rehabilitation. | Adult day care centers—Activity programs.
Classification: LCC RC521 .W628 2020 | DDC 616.8/31—dc23
LC record available at https://lccn.loc.gov/2019023261

A catalog record for this book is available from the British Library.

The image on page 8 is adapted from R. Wonderlin, *When Someone You Know Is Living in a Dementia Care Community*, Baltimore, MD, Johns Hopkins University Press, 2016. All other images are © iStockphoto.com unless otherwise noted.

Special discounts are available for bulk purchases of this book. For more information, please contact Special Sales at specialsales@press.jhu.edu.

Johns Hopkins University Press uses environmentally friendly book materials, including recycled text paper that is composed of at least 30 percent post-consumer waste, whenever possible.

For David, for all your love and support

Contents

PART III

ACTIVITIES

Creative Engagement

What Are Dementia-Friendly Activities?

When we talk about "dementia-friendly" environments or activities, we are talking about items that meet the physical and emotional needs of adults living with dementia. One of my main goals when creating dementia-friendly activities is to offer ways to engage adults with dementia that is fun and challenging but not childish. We want to be able to live in the world of the person with dementia rather than trying to drag them into ours.

The goal of this book is to provide ideas for activities that you can do with your loved one or resident who has dementia. As I wrote this, I kept in mind activity directors, recreation therapists, families, professional caregivers, dementia care directors, and more. I have worked in a number of different care communities, and I have always noticed the same thing: activities are the lifeblood of a dementia care environment. The community can be beautiful, clean, and full of residents, but when those residents have nothing to do, the environment is severely lacking. Bored residents are unhappy residents. Bored residents will also fall more often, get into more arguments, become depressed, eat less, and overall enjoy life less. The happiest communities that I have seen are ones that have full, engaging activity calendars. The staff is happier, the residents are happier, and the residents' families are happier.

Creative engagement is one of the organizing principles that caregivers need to keep in mind when planning activities for someone with dementia. Although it is a cliché that every person is different, it's important to remember that dementia is different in every person in terms of severity, in terms of the person's history, and so forth. We cannot state too often that the type of activities that work with one person may not be appropriate for another. Care partners must be creative in their approaches, trying out different options, seeing what works and what doesn't, talking to others, learning, and constantly customizing. Although this approach does require work upfront and continual assessment, the payoff in terms of engagement, in terms of improved communication, in terms of better relationships, is worth it. I'd like to hear from you with your stories of "creative engagement." Please email Rachael at rachael@dementiabyday.com.

The same concept works at home. Just because someone with dementia lives at home does not mean that they are inherently happier than someone who lives in a care community. I have often heard caregiver children say that "the reason they do not want to move their parent into a care community is because their parent loves being at home." While Mom or Dad may love home, if they have nothing to do there, they will become just as depressed and bored as someone who lives in a boring care community.

In many of the chapters that follow I offer activities for those in a community setting as well as those at home. I recommend reading both sections, even if your loved one lives at home and won't be moving or even if you work in senior housing and don't intend on switching to home care. I share stories from both sides of the aisle because that may help you when creating a new activity or if you do eventually consider relocating a loved one.

There is much research looking at best practices for caring for a loved one with dementia. Scholars in the fields of psychology, social work, gerontology, nursing, occupational therapy, and even environmental gerontology have researched quality care and activities. So while I speak from experience, I am grateful that the scientific community is helping us all develop a greater understanding of what works, and sometimes what does *not* work, in caring for persons living with dementia from all walks of life. When relevant, I cite these sources as well.

Daily engagement is much more than just a nice activity calendar and a good activity staff. It's about the lifestyle that you offer inside of your house or at a senior living community. From morning to night, adults with dementia should be offered a life that is interesting, fun, and similar to the one that they always lived. No one wants to feel as though their life is unimportant or inconsequential. It is our job, as caregivers, to provide people with dementia with an opportunity to continue living a life worth living.

PART I

BACKGROUND

What Is Dementia?

Before we begin talking about activities for people with dementia, we need to first review what dementia is. While many people work with loved ones or clients who have dementia, they may not necessarily be able to describe what the term "dementia" actually means. *Dementia is a group of symptoms that can be caused by many diseases and causes cognitive loss over time* (Mace & Rabins, 2017). This can be a confusing definition: what does cognitive loss over time mean? Isn't dementia just another form of Alzheimer disease? No, and here's how I often explain it: when I describe dementia, I talk about it the way we talk about cancer. For example, if you were to go to the doctor and the doctor told you that you had cancer, you wouldn't say, "Okay, thanks," and then leave. You would probably ask, "What type of cancer is it?" This likewise applies when a doctor says your loved one has dementia. You should ask the doctor, "What form of dementia is it?" Unfortunately, most people leave the physician's office with more questions than they went in with. They do not know to ask about the cause of the dementia, assume it means "something to do with memory loss," and head out the door.

"Dementia" is an umbrella term (figure 1.1), much like cancer is an umbrella term. There are more than seventy different causes of dementia. I have had people say things to me like "I know what Alzheimer's is, but what is dementia?" They assume because the two words are often used in the same sentence that they are different things. But just as "cancer" is the umbrella term and breast cancer is the specific type of cancer, so "dementia" is the umbrella term, and Alzheimer disease is the specific cause or form of dementia.

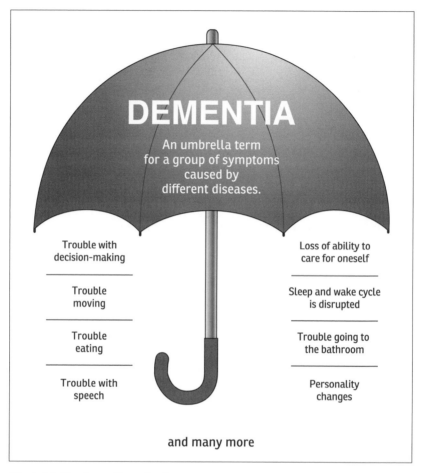

Figure 1.1. The dementia umbrella

When people think about dementia, they connect it with memory loss. But not everyone with dementia has a memory problem, and memory problems are not the only symptom of dementia. Any symptom that falls under the category of cognitive loss, such as spatial awareness challenges, mood changes, paranoia, confusion, irritability, aphasia, and, of course, memory loss, can be a symptom of dementia. For example, a brain tumor could be considered a cause of dementia. We are also seeing a lot more people with CTE (chronic traumatic encephalopathy), a degenerative brain disease that often is tied to recurring concussions, developing dementia later in life. Alcoholic dementia is another form of cognitive loss people do not often think about. Wernicke-Korsakoff syndrome is a vitamin B1 (thiamine) deficiency, often caused by severe and long-term alcoholism, that may produce symptoms of dementia such as confusion and memory problems (Budson & Kowall, 2014).

The four most common causes of dementia are Alzheimer disease, vascular dementia, dementia with Lewy bodies, and frontotemporal lobar dementia. For the purpose of this book, we don't need to go into great detail for each type of dementia, but I do review a few symptoms for each of these dementias.

ALZHEIMER DISEASE

While there are other symptoms, the prevailing symptom of Alzheimer disease is short-term memory challenges that get progressively worse. People with Alzheimer's have a lot of trouble remembering what they ate for breakfast, what they did yesterday, or, in later stages, recalling the information you told them just minutes ago. People with Alzheimer's also experience some mood changes and paranoia, especially in earlier stages of the disease. It's important to make a distinction between early-onset or younger-onset Alzheimer disease and later-onset Alzheimer disease. Early-onset disease is diagnosed in individuals who are younger than 65. It is also very heritable, which means that first-degree relatives of someone with early-onset have a significant chance of also getting the disorder, and genetic testing can often detect the gene mutations most likely to cause the disease. Unlike later-onset Alzheimer disease, early-onset memory loss progresses more rapidly. Recently I have heard people use the terms "early onset" and "early stage" interchangeably. But they should not be used interchangeably, because they do not mean the same thing: "early onset" means the disease appears before a person's mid-60s, while "early stage" just means that a person is in the beginning part of the disease process. Some profession-als are beginning to use the term "younger onset" in order to clarify the difference between the terms (Mace & Rabins, 2017).

VASCULAR DEMENTIA

Another common form of dementia is vascular dementia, which many people used to call a "hardening of the arteries." Vascular dementia is caused by cardiovascular issues like strokes, diabetes, obesity, chronic heart failure, and more. People with vascular dementia do have short-term memory troubles, but they are typically not as pronounced as in someone with Alzheimer disease. They will often have issues with gait impairment and visual/spatial awareness (Budson & Kowall, 2014). I have noticed that while many people living with Alzheimer's are up, walking with ease, many people with vascular dementia are in wheel-chairs or relying on walkers.

DEMENTIA WITH LEWY BODIES

Dementia with Lewy bodies (DLB) is a progressive form of dementia in which individuals may have visual hallucinations, symptoms similar to Parkinson disease, cognitive problems, sleep problems, depression, and apathy. In other words, a cluster of cognitive, behavioral, and emotional challenges. Lewy body *diseases* encompass three diseases: Parkinson disease, Parkinson disease dementia, and DLB. One can have Parkinson's and not get dementia, or one can have Parkinson's and then get demen-tia later on in the disease process. People with DLB often have some Par-kinsonian symptoms, although they lack full-blown Parkinson's. DLB is often harder than Alzheimer's or vascular dementia for caregivers to cope with for two reasons: people with DLB tend to hallucinate, and they have what is called "fluctuating impairment." Hallucinations are different from delusions, which are fixed false ideas. Hallucinations are when a person is seeing or hearing something that is not there. Fluctuating impairment refers to a disease process in which a person's impairment changes throughout the week. Some days, people with DLB are very "with it," while other days, they are very confused and disoriented. It can be challenging to predict which days will be harder than others and therefore difficult for many caregivers to cope with (Budson & Kowall, 2014).

FRONTOTEMPORAL LOBAR DEMENTIA

The final form of dementia that we review in any detail is frontotemporal lobar dementia (FTD). FTD tends to affect people who are younger, typically between the ages of 45 and 65. It can occur in older adults, as well, although the fact that more of those affected are younger often makes it more challenging for families to deal with. People with FTD may display a lot of behavioral problems that also make the disease very difficult. The disease affects the frontal and temporal lobes of the brain, which are the filter, planning, and decision-making parts, or executive functions, of the brain. People with FTD tend to be very impulsive, lack the ability to plan or make healthy choices, and often lack a "filter," so they will say and do awkward or socially inappropriate things. People with FTD may do or say sexually inappropriate things as well, which makes it uncomfortable for family members who are taking care of them. Adults with FTD often do not live successfully in care community settings: they are often much younger, more mobile, and more disinhibited than other residents in the community (Mace & Rabins, 2017).

DOES IT MATTER WHAT FORM
OF DEMENTIA IT IS?

Often, I am asked, "Is it important to know what form of dementia my loved one has?" I usually tell people that, yes, it is important to know what type of dementia a loved one has. You want to know what to expect and when you should seek medical treatment for someone. For example, if your mother has Alzheimer disease and is hallucinating, you will want to get her checked for a urinary tract infection, which is the most common cause of delirium (a sudden onset of confusion). If your mother has a diagnosis of DLB, though, and she is hallucinating, this is probably normal for her and does not need to be dealt with immediately, since hallucinations are part of the DLB disease process.

This chapter is not intended to be a detailed description of the different forms of dementia, but I hope it gets you to think about how the way the disease is treated depends on the symptoms of different causes of dementia. *The 36-Hour Day*, written by Nancy L. Mace and Dr. Peter V. Rabins, was first published by Johns Hopkins University Press over thirty years ago. It is currently in its sixth edition and includes detailed descriptions of many causes of dementia. You might want to go to the Alzheimer's Association webpage (alz.org) and check out my first book, *When Someone You Know Is Living in a Dementia Care Community* (also published by Johns Hopkins University Press). There you'll find much more information about dementia and even some of the current research being done to find a cure for Alzheimer disease.

2

Building a Dementia-Friendly Environment

The skilled nursing facility's dementia care unit was nothing to write home about. It smelled fine and was generally clean, but it was boring. Residents hung out in the dining room even when it was not mealtime. No one would have known that it was a dementia care wing, because it did not look different from any other space in the building. The first thing that I did when I got there was open up the box of a brand-new CD player I had purchased. I put the CD player on a small table in the hallway. The second the music came on, residents began to gather around. I moved a few chairs closer to the music. Within the next half hour, residents were practically fighting each other to sit near the CD player. All it took was some music and some furniture rearranging, but the space felt completely different.

Dementia-friendly interior design is, oddly enough, a fairly new concept. When you go into a senior care community, you typically find one of two things: it is either designed with family members in mind, or it looks like a hurricane hit. It's either beautiful and clean but stark and boring, or it's dirty, disorganized, and confusing—and sometimes it is both. While I have seen beautiful, dementia-friendly design, it is rare.

Dementia-friendly design aspects can be used at home, as well. You don't need to paint walls or completely rearrange rooms to create a dementia-positive space, either. For the majority of this chapter, I discuss dementia-friendly design in a community-based setting, but these design aspects can work at home as well.

It has been suggested that people who have dementia are even more dependent on the environment in which they're living than people without dementia, something called the environmental press theory (Lawton, 1983). People with dementia have fewer cognitive resources that they can draw on to cope with the environment they find themselves in. If someone without dementia is living in a place where there are no activities—or no activities they enjoy—or where they do not find the company of those they are living with pleasurable, they have the resources to find those activities and those people that *do* make them happy. Thus it is imperative that the living environment for those with dementia, and without the cognitive resources to change things, be dementia-friendly.

Dementia-friendly design is as much a part of daily activity engagement as having a great activity director who runs regular programming. If your home or care community is not environmentally dementia-friendly, it cannot be truly dementia-friendly from a programming standpoint. These things go hand in hand.

When you walk into a dementia care community, you should feel that it is different from the rest of the building. It should feel like you are walking into a different world: a world where people living with dementia can thrive and enjoy their lives. The same thing goes for a house where someone with dementia lives: it will have to look and feel different if it is to meet the needs of the resident with dementia.

IN A COMMUNITY SETTING

In a dementia care community setting, the environment needs to match the needs of the residents with dementia. It is not enough to have a community with a great activity calendar—it should also offer a great physical space that matches the world that the residents live in. As we

know, many people with dementia live in the past. My best recommen-
dation, always, is to create an environment that matches that world
instead of trying to thrust people with dementia into the present or
future.

We want to offer a world to our residents that they recognize. Instead of having a basic nurses' station at the entrance to the community,
we have a soda fountain counter. Sure, it functions as a nurses' station
(the nurses can work behind the counter) but the residents are able to
sit at the "soda counter" and enjoy a beverage while they listen to music
or get their medicine. For some people who grew up in the 1940s and
1950s, soda fountain counters were a normal part of daily life. We want
to cater to the group of residents that live in that community. There is
no reason that a functional piece in a dementia care community can't
also be creative and beautiful.

We can have spaces where residents can work that contain a desk
complete with a computer, a planner, and pencils. We can offer a nursery for baby dolls, a dresser full of clothes to try on and fold, a space for
stuffed animals that look and feel real. There are so many creative options that come to mind when designing an interactive space for people
living with dementia.

What you see a lot of are places that cater to residents' families'
needs and desires. I cannot tell you how many communities that I have
gone to where the dementia care wing looks like a hotel. A nice hotel,
but a hotel, nonetheless. The ceilings are high, the chairs are cushioned,
and a glass chandelier hangs near the entrance. Places like these are not
made for residents with dementia: they are made to make you want to
pay for your loved one to live there. They are built to assuage your guilt.
They are made so that you can tell your next-door neighbor, "Mom is in
a great place! They have a really nice chandelier up front. It's so beautiful." Just because a place is beautiful does not mean that it is functional
or good or that it has been created with people with cognitive impairments in mind. I am not saying that a place with a modern look cannot
be dementia-friendly, but what I am suggesting is that most people

with dementia did not grow up in homes that look like they were built in 2020. Steel countertops, rustic furniture, and wrought-iron handles on cabinetry look nice, but if a resident does not know what something is used for, they will not use it. If your community's communal kitchen has a sink that looks like it was made in the year 3000, your residents might not even know that it's a sink.

A lot of well-meaning communities have begun to rely on technology to care for people living with dementia. You may find that there are interactive computer programs for residents to use or even a Nintendo Wii bowling game set up. These items are great for people without dementia, but what I have often found is that adults with dementia have a really hard time understanding what these technology programs are or how to use them. This is the same reason why you will not often see residents with dementia use call buttons in their rooms: they don't know that the call button is an option. While fancy tech often makes families feel better (e.g., "Mom's community gives everyone iPads!") it does not typically make the lives of the residents any better. It is one thing if the staff is able to integrate technology to use with residents, but is a problem if residents are expected to use it by themselves.

Furniture and Patterns

So many care communities do not think correctly about decor for their residents with dementia. They are looking for what looks good instead of what is actually most functional for people with dementia. I cannot tell you how many times I've seen colorful, patterned chairs with no armrests. While these types of options for furniture look nice, they are not practical in a dementia care environment. For one, patterns are often confusing for people living with dementia. They will reach for and try to pick up the leaves from a leaf-patterned fabric on a chair, because the one-dimensional pattern looks real to them. Further, fabric in general is impractical for chairs and couches in dementia care communities. Fabrics are hard to clean and wipe off. If someone has a bathroom accident on a fabric chair, that chair is ruined. If that chair was made out of vinyl, though, the housekeeping staff could wipe it down. A good example of a chair that could work in a care community is shown in figure 2.1. Care communities get a lot more mileage out of furniture that is washable!

I had a resident once who would constantly try to pick the lines off the carpeted floor. When Betty got particularly confused, she'd spend hours bending down and practically falling over trying to peel lines off the carpet. Not only was the carpet a safety hazard for our residents but it was also impractical, as it got stained and dirty far too quickly. The community had purchased it because it was softer than hardwood flooring, but the downsides of the carpet outweighed its softness. Environment is as important as activities and engagement in creating a great space for residents.

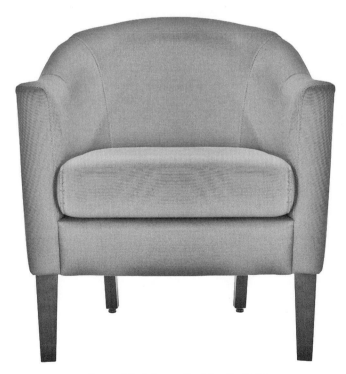

Figure 2.1. A dementia-friendly chair

Use of Baby Dolls and Stuffed Animals

One of my favorite things to set up in a care community is what I call the "nursery station" (figure 2.2). It's an interactive space where residents can come and go as they please. I've often made up a whole room to look like a baby's nursery. There are realistic-looking baby dolls lying down and sitting up in a real crib. Nursery decor lines the walls, and there is pleasant music on repeat in the corner, drawing attention to the space. The door to the room is always kept open, or we take the door off. The warm wall colors, music, and details in the space encourage residents to enter the nursery. A couple rocking chairs are set up so that residents can take the babies out and sit with them. There are baby clothes in a basket, and baby socks waiting to be matched.

I have found that some of the best activities for people with dementia are those that require little to no involvement of the staff. People living with dementia are prone to walking or wheeling up and down the halls looking for things to do. For the person who stumbles on a

Figure 2.2. Interactive spaces increase engagement with realistic-looking dolls

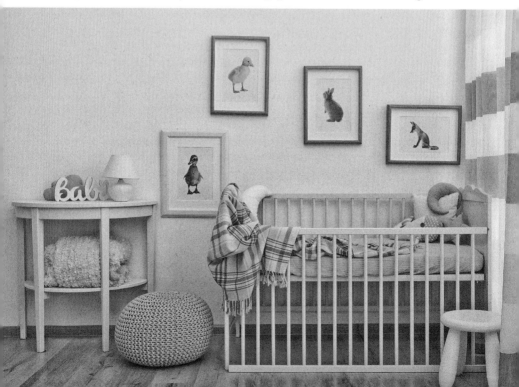

nursery, particularly when they believe that the babies are real, it is a beautiful find. I have seen residents' whole days turn around just by holding a baby doll.

When I don't know if a resident will think a baby doll is real or not, I offer it to them by asking, "What do you think about this?" I know right away if the resident believes the baby is real or not, based on their reaction. If they say, "Oh! A baby!" I say, "Yes, a baby." If they say, "Oh! It's a cute doll," I say, "Yes, it's a cute doll." In either case, I allow the resident to tell me what the doll is, and then I agree with what they say. To help people with dementia, you need to set a happy tone and create a pleasant environment and then back away and let the people with dementia guide you.

When it comes to stuffed animals, I do the same thing. I set up a space that looks like a pet shop or else just put a raised table with a pet bed on it in a room. I set up realistic-looking animals and let them be, returning only to set them back up or wash them. I let the residents at the community guide me. What do they like? What do they want? I take these clues and live in their world. More on this in a later chapter.

A Workspace

Probably the best thing about this space is that it requires very little setup. A desk, a computer, a calendar on the wall, and a cup of pencils can easily create the feel of a workspace. I've often created "workspaces" for residents that contain a desk that resembles one they used to have in their home or at their office. For my residents who believe that they are still going to work every day, this is a welcome sight. I like to ask them to "help me" finish a project or plan for an upcoming event. I once had a retired wedding planner as a resident, and he was a great fit for this space. I'd put him on a project for an upcoming event and he would sit for quite a while, reviewing his plans.

Dining Space

When creating a dining space for people with dementia, I look to design a warm, inviting area that encourages eating and communication. After all, that's what you would want in a kitchen at home or a restaurant out with friends. I love themes, so when I consult with a dementia care community I try to make the kitchen look like something, be it a 1950s-style kitchen, a restaurant, or a coffee shop. I want people to feel comfortable, happy, and lively while they are there.

One thing that I always include in a dining space is a large menu board. Residents who like to read always look to the menu to see what's being served that day. It provides them with a sense of comfort to know what is coming up next and not just have a plate set in front of them. I always ensure that music is playing while the residents eat as well. Plates work best when they aren't too heavy, aren't breakable, and are a bright color, like red. Residents should be able to tell the difference between the plate and the food that is on it.

If possible, dining areas and activity areas should be separate. I have been to many communities where the activity space and the dining space are shared, and this is a challenge. When a meal ends, everyone scrambles to clean up and set up the next activity. Residents also associate the activity space with food or the food space with activities. I think it is best to create a space that is separate, so that it has a distinct identity that resonates with the residents and staff.

AT HOME

We sat at Garrett's kitchen table, discussing what their daily activities included. Garrett was taking care of his father in his house, but he regularly hired caregivers to come in and help while he was at work. I had come to meet Pete and do an assessment, and Garrett pored through his daily schedule and notes with me. "You see," he said, "here I have his daily checklist, which the caregivers check off, and here's where we write down his exercises, and here's where they sign off that he brushed his teeth for a full sixty seconds!" Garrett smiled. He had everything down to a science—or so he thought. Pete had a lot of trouble walking, and he didn't have much space to walk in. His walker took up the entire hallway, and he was not a small man. Pete was also expected to step into his claw-foot tub without much assistance. "Dad has an alert necklace," Garrett explained. "He can press that if he falls and no one is here." My heart sank. "Garrett," I said. "He's not going to press that if he falls. He has no idea what that necklace is even for." "Sure he does!" he said. "Hey, Dad, what would you do if you fell?" Pete looked up from the paper he was looking at, but perhaps not reading. "Well," he said, slowly. "I suppose I'd . . . yell very loudly for help!" He smiled, proud that he had found an answer. Garrett shook his head. "But Dad . . . what about that necklace on your neck?" he said, pointing to the necklace that his father had forgotten he was wearing. Pete looked down at it, looked back up at Garrett, and shrugged. "Would you . . . press it for help?" Garrett said slowly. "Yes, I would press it for help," Pete parroted back. "See, he knows," Garrett said, kind of smugly.

"Garrett," I said, "he can parrot back what you say all day, but he's never going to press that."

There was no way that Pete was going to know how to help himself if he fell. He was a sweet, confused man who spent many of his hours alone. It was a terrible accident waiting to happen. The house was not equipped for a 250 lb, 85-year-old man with dementia. There was clutter everywhere, too many pieces of furniture, and not enough walking space. Pete was in serious danger, especially without someone there twenty-four hours a day, seven days a week.

Garrett had made a terrible error in judgment: he was relying on technology to keep his father safe. He had assumed that an alert necklace would protect him as well as would a person hired to undertake twenty-four-hour care, and that just wasn't true. Technology, at least at this time, cannot replace human care when it comes to dementia.

My rule is this: if your loved one has dementia, they should never be at home alone. Even in an early stage of impairment, things can go wrong very, very quickly. Just because Dad has been living at home by himself for twenty years does not mean he can keep doing that now that he has dementia. Patterns one has followed for twenty years can go right out the window when someone is confused or lost.

Making Home Safe

How do you make your home safe for someone with dementia? Here is a basic, easy-to-follow checklist that will help you succeed with having your loved one at home:

- Twenty-four-hour care: you can have the best, most well-equipped home in the world, but unless another human being is there to care for your loved one with dementia, it will not matter.

- Space to get around: you do not want a ton of furniture and tables clogging the way, especially if your loved one has a walker or wheelchair.

- No throw rugs: you do not want rugs that can lift easily and cause slipping or tripping.

- Nothing black on the floor: many people with dementia perceive black rugs on the floor as holes.

- Minimal stairs or steps.

- A walk-in tub, not a step-over tub.

- Plenty of lighting: you do not want dark corners or stairs.

- Minimal patterns on furniture: some patterns on furniture can look real (e.g., leaves, which people with dementia might try to pick off your cushioned living room chair).

- Warm colors on walls: you do not want bright, wild colors, but you also do not want dark, hard to see paints either.

- Hand rails: you want a hand rail near the toilet, one near the bed, and some on the stairs.

Your loved one can be safe at home if they are not left alone. Also, if you have a large house with a lot of stairs that you don't want your loved one going down, "making rules" will not help you. Telling Dad that he "isn't allowed" to go down to the basement is not going to stop him from going down to the basement if he wants to do so. Ensuring that the people that are caring for your loved one are capable and that the type of home that they are living in is well designed is critical to keeping them safe at home.

Baby Dolls and Stuffed Animals

I love using baby dolls and stuffed animals in dementia care. I use them constantly in dementia care communities, and I have seen them work beautifully in home care situations as well. There is no reason that you cannot set up a "nursery" or "pet station" in your house. All it takes is a small space and a couple of items.

The key when choosing a baby or stuffed animal for your loved one is to take a moment to try it out. Present the baby to your loved one and say, "What do you think about this?" This will give your loved one an opportunity to tell you if they think it is real or not. If they believe the baby is real, it is real. If they believe that the baby is not real, it is not real. Either answer is correct, and do not try to force a belief onto a loved one who does not react the way you'd like.

If you want to get a baby doll for your loved one, spend a few extra dollars and pick up a bassinet for the baby to sleep in. Designate a spot in the house for the baby to stay in and put the baby doll back there each night. This will save you a lot of pain and effort when your loved one needs to go to sleep and wants to take the baby with them to bed. It will also help you when they are more focused on "getting the baby something to eat." All you need to do during these times is to say, "I think the baby needs a nap," and take it to the bassinet. If your loved one is prone to losing things (and most people with dementia are) pick up a couple copies of the baby and put them in a closet. When baby goes missing, you will not have a meltdown on your hands: you will have a backup baby ready to go.

If you want a stuffed animal that looks real for your loved one, designate a space in the house for a pet bed. Get a dog bed from a local pet store and set that in a room where the pet will stay when it is not with your loved one. Employ the technique of, "I'll put the dog down for a nap," when you want your loved one to focus attention elsewhere. As I recommend with the baby dolls, have a backup pet or two in case the first one goes missing (figure 2.3).

Other Creative Spaces

Think about what your loved one enjoyed doing when they didn't have dementia. Did they value a productive workday at the office? Did they spend most of their time cleaning the house? Did they raise children or care for animals? Incorporate what you know about your loved one into the physical space. For example, someone who worked and valued work will probably enjoy the opportunity to continue doing just that. Set up a desk and a computer, and give them an important task to complete (even if you have to make up a task for this to work). If they loved tinkering and building, save a space for this. Make an area where they can work with their hands all day if they so choose.

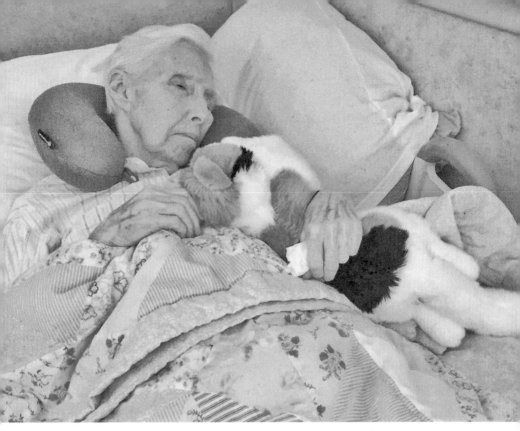

Figure 2.3. Have a backup stuffed animal in case something happens to the first one. Used with permission of MemorablePets.com.

Dining Space

In dementia care communities, the daily calendar provides a structure for when breakfast, lunch and dinner are offered. In home care, however, there is often no overarching plan for meals. I recommend that you do establish a certain time and designate a certain space for meals; do not get in the habit of serving your loved one frozen dinners as they sit in front of a TV. Make a space at the dining room table for meals, and stick to using that space. Your loved one with dementia will eventually begin to associate that space with eating, so it will be easier to get them to eat when they sit in that area.

Have a couple choices available, but do not offer too many. Opening the fridge and saying, "What do you want to eat?" is only going to cause confusion and frustration for both of you. That opens the door to way too many choices. Instead, offer two choices of meal options. The other thing that you may want to do is to create a menu for each week. While it may take more time in the beginning, you may find that it saves you time later on.

SUMMING IT ALL UP

Creating a dementia-friendly environment is as much about physical space as it is about activities. Environment is the foundation that you build on, and if the foundation isn't strong, the rest of your activity programming won't be either. Be it at home or in a care community, adults with dementia need spaces that cater to their emotional and physical needs. Creating that kind of space will give you a lot more flexibility and freedom going forward. It also saves you from having to entertain your loved one or resident with dementia all day, because they have spaces to occupy their time. They can take care of a baby doll, spend time in the garden, or relax in a comfortable chair in the living room. These all count as activities, because they are all meaningful to the person with dementia.

3

Caregiver Stress

Dan found me after class one day. I'd been teaching at a local university in an older-adult learning program. Dan had taken my class the semester before and had been struggling with his father's care. He and his wife had been keeping his father, Jonathan, at their house while he healed after hip surgery, but the caregiving was becoming too much to bear. Jonathan's dementia was progressing, and so was his poor mood. The husband-and-wife duo took turns staying home with Jon so that he would be safe. They took turns getting up in the middle of the night to care for him when he woke up to use the bathroom. They took turns taking Jon to his doctors' appointments, making sure he ate and bathed, and generally caring for him, twenty-four hours a day, seven days a week.

Not surprisingly, this took a deep toll on the couple's life. Although they were both retired, they had previously been quite busy during the day. Now, with the concern and constant care for Jon's life, Dan and his wife were unable to leave the house for very long at all. It put undue stress on them as individuals and on their previously happy relationship. Now, they fought over the silliest things. Dan and his wife had raised two children together—they assumed that caring for his father would be a snap!

Dan had bought my book and attended each class of the course I had been teaching, sitting dutifully in the front row, taking notes. At the end of the course, he had asked me for some advice. "I love my father," he said, "but the man is driving me insane. I don't know what to do. You talked a lot about where someone with dementia could live, and my wife and I are considering moving him to an assisted living community around here. Do you have any recommendations?" I recommended a community that I had a personal connection with and trusted. Dan visited the community I recommended, signed the paperwork, and moved his father there the next week.

Now, he'd found me after class again and wanted to tell me about his experience. "I can't tell you how personally indebted I am to you," he said. "My dad is doing so well at his new home. The staff is excellent, he's engaged in activities, he goes on outings . . . I actually think he's improved. I can't tell you how happy we are that we moved him. It's such a relief to know that he's safe and well cared for." Hearing this from my former student brought tears to my eyes. You could hear the pure relief in his voice: he didn't even need to say it. Dan's father was being taken care of around the clock, and the couple was freed from the stress of worrying, rushing around, and providing twenty-four-hour care.

IT'S NOT LIKE CARING FOR A CHILD

As caregivers often come to find, caring for someone with dementia is much different, and oftentimes much more difficult, than caring for a healthy child. After speaking to hundreds, if not thousands, of caregivers, I can tell you that they all feel the same thing: guilt. Caregivers feel as though they need to be their loved ones' constant companion and caregiver and do not immediately recognize the weight that they must shoulder to be able to provide around-the-clock care. Caring for children is, no doubt, a stressful endeavor. However, healthy children continue to grow and develop. They learn new things, they begin to do more for themselves, and they begin to develop lives of their own. Adults with dementia are the complete opposite: they are growing sicker, they are growing weaker, and they are losing the gains they've made as adults. We do not care for people with dementia with the expectation that they will recover or get better. Instead, we care for them with the hope of maintaining a certain baseline; we aim to ensure that they remain strong and independent for as long as possible, all the while knowing that they will continue to decline.

There is also the added stress that people with dementia are adults. They have lived full lives and often do not take kindly to being "bossed around" or being told what to do, especially by their adult children. People with dementia come into the disease process with years of life experience, and when we suddenly take privileges away from them, such as driving a car, it can cause a lot of friction. Taking privileges away from children is completely different, because as a parent or adult figure, you are expected to do that. Taking things from people with dementia is much harder because they do not expect it. Caregivers are tasked with the impossible: care for this person, worry about this person, feed, clothe, bathe, plan for this person, and ensure that they are behaviorally, physically, and emotionally stable and healthy. When an adult with dementia is in a near-constant state of decline, for every step that you take in providing the best care, the adult with dementia you are caring for essentially takes two steps back. The disease is always a step ahead of the caregiver.

GUILT

Quite often, I meet caregivers who, like Dan and his wife, have begun to miss out on other aspects of life because of the care they are providing to their loved one. Caregiving quickly takes on a life of its own, and caregivers may find themselves without many coping mechanisms or strategies. They refuse to set aside time to have lunch with a friend or go see a movie, punishing themselves because they feel as though they must shoulder the entire weight of the caregiving burden. This is not fair for the caregiver, and it really is not fair for the person with dementia either.

One of the main reasons that I wrote my first book, *When Someone You Know is Living in a Dementia Care Community*, was because I
wanted to reach caregivers who felt that they had no options. I met
many caregivers who felt they had no choice but to assume full care
of their ailing loved one at home. They felt as though there was nowhere else to turn, that a dementia care community was not an option
owing to the stigma surrounding such communities. I usually heard
things like "I don't want to move Mom into a nursing home, that's just
like prison" or "I can't hire extra help for my husband with dementia. I don't trust anyone else to take care of him." While many caregivers may feel this way, the fact is that such sentiments only perpetuate
the vicious cycle of being someone's sole caregiver. A lot of the time,
it's the guilt talking. Somewhere along the line, a loved one with dementia said, "Don't ever put me in a home" or "Just kill me if I start to
lose my memory!" Statements like these make caregivers feel guilty
and responsible. They don't want to let their loved ones with dementia
down, so they shoulder the full weight of caregiving. Caregiver guilt is
even recognized by psychologists. In 2010, a questionnaire was developed regarding caregiver guilt. Sure enough, being female and caring
for a parent with dementia were associated with higher levels of guilt
(Losada, Márquez-González, Puente, & Romero-Moreno, 2010). The
questionnaire asks about different types of guilt experienced by caregivers such as feeling guilty about doing "wrong" by the care receiver,
failing to meet the challenges of caregiving, experiencing negative
emotions about caregiving, not taking care of oneself, and neglect-
ing other relatives (Roach, Laidlaw, Gillanders, & Quinn, 2013). Because of the emotional and physical toll that caregiving takes, it ends
up not benefiting the person with dementia. It's not uncommon for
me to walk into a client's house and see that the adult daughter has
composed hundreds of notes for the person with dementia. Things like
"Dad, you live here now, don't go outside" or "Dad, you have a memory
problem, remember?" I usually try to find a way to tell the family that
these notes don't help and often make the person with dementia feel

worse. I also keep in mind, however, that these notes were written out of both love and guilt. Caregivers think that if they cannot be with the person with dementia twenty-four seven, then if they create notes such as these there will at least be information left to keep the person safe. However, these notes don't work. Typically, people with dementia don't even know to read them. The immense weight of caregiving results in the caregiver worrying constantly about their loved one's safety. Even if the caregiver is away from their loved one, they remain worried and distracted, thinking about the person with dementia.

THE PHYSICAL AND EMOTIONAL TOLL OF STRESS

A few years ago I watched a video of the 1995 Glaser experiment in which caregivers of patients with dementia and other people the same ages as the caregivers were administered small "punch biopsy" wounds, and then the time it took for the wounds to heal was photographed. Sure enough, the wounds on the caregivers of dementia patients took longer to heal than those of the noncaregiving comparison group. This was my introduction to the impact of caregiving on the physical health of caregivers.

Much has been written about how stress impacts the body, and caregiving is quite stressful. Some even call caregivers of someone with dementia a "second patient" because of the toll it can take on the body. The Glaser experiment was designed to examine the impact of caregiving on the immune systems of caregivers, and the conclusion was that owing to the stress of caregiving, they have a harder time healing from illnesses such as colds and other infections (Kiecolt-Glaser, Glaser, Gravenstein, Malarkey, & Sheridan, 1996). Caregivers often talk about extreme fatigue and sleeplessness; they tend to spend time they should be sleeping giving attention to, or worrying about, their loved one with dementia. Caregivers often forget to eat or eat on the run while attending to their loved one. There is also a strong connection between stress and intestinal problems, particularly constipation. Still other caregivers share that they have a hard time even concentrating on things they're trying to accomplish or even on things like hobbies and other activities that they used to enjoy. In worse case scenarios, some caregivers turn to drugs and alcohol to cope.

But the stress of caregiving also impacts caregivers emotionally. The anxiety and worry associated with caregiving is oftentimes the reason for sleep and eating problems. Although caregivers need support and should spend time with others, many share that they are just far too busy to stay involved with friends and activities that were important to them. So the cycle begins. Caregivers are exhausted and feel that they don't have time to spend with their friends and other loved ones, so they withdraw. The more they withdraw, the more they begin to feel that they have nothing to even contribute to their friendships—they don't want to take their friends' time and just vent about their caregiving—so they withdraw even further, which leads to even more distress and frustration at being so isolated from others. The American Medical Association has even created a questionnaire to help caregivers evaluate their own well-being. It aims to help caregivers begin to see how the stress is affecting them by asking questions about whether they feel overwhelmed, lonely, or irritable.

A BETTER OPTION

Here is the good news: you have other options. When I host workshops for caregivers, I always start with a question. "Who here is their loved one's sole caregiver?" I ask. Most everyone raises their hand. "Okay," I tell them. "I want all of you to stop being your loved one's sole caregiver as soon as possible." Everyone laughs anxiously, unsure of what I mean. It is almost as though the thought that they could stop being the only caregiver hadn't occurred to anyone in the room.

Not only is attempting to shoulder the caregiving burden unfair to you and your loved one, it is also irresponsible! It is not possible to be someone's everything all of the time. That we have adult day care, respite care, professional caregivers, home care agencies, skilled nursing facilities, and assisted living communities means you don't have to try to be everything all the time. At long-term care communities, there is an entire team of individuals responsible for caring for your loved one around the clock.

Natalie was her mother's sole caregiver. I liked Natalie a lot, and she was clearly devoted to learning as much about dementia as she possibly could. She attended every workshop and class that I offered within a thirty-mile radius of Pittsburgh, and she always had a notebook in which she took diligent notes. Every time I saw Natalie, she'd tell me how exhausted she was. After seeing her a number of times in this state of exhaustion I finally asked, "When are you going to change your caregiving circumstances?" She was taken aback. "What do you mean?" she asked. "There's no one else to take care of my mom!" "That's not true," I explained. "You have a lot of options, but your guilt isn't letting you choose anything else." Natalie burst into tears. "You're right," she replied, sighing.

I check in with Natalie every so often. As far as I know, she's still her mother's sole caregiver. For the sake of both herself and her mother, I want Natalie to stop harboring so much guilt. I hope that someday soon, she will choose to hire a home care agency, move her mother to assisted living, or bring her mom to an adult day care facility, even just twice a week. I don't think that Natalie is going to do any of these things, though. She feels too responsible, too guilty, and too anxious to move forward with a plan.

For all the caregivers out there: there are a lot of options for your loved one's safe and secure care, so release yourself from guilt. You can still be a wonderful caregiver, even if you aren't with your loved one constantly. In fact, I have often found that the happiest caregivers are ones who are not beside their loved ones with dementia around the clock. Do yourself a favor, and do your loved one a favor: shoulder less of the caregiving burden.

PART II

TIPS

4

Creating a Calendar

Both home caregivers and care communities often forego calendars. Typically, the excuse for not creating a calendar is that people with dementia don't read it. However, even if they do not read the engagement calendar, many still rely on daily patterns for clues about when it is time to eat, start a new activity, or go to sleep.

Calendars also provide a way for caregivers (both professional and family caregivers) to schedule a predictable day. Without a plan, providing care for a person with dementia can be overwhelming. Further, many caregivers find that having no plan is equivalent to having a dull, open-ended day. People with dementia lack the ability to plan ahead, so the impetus falls entirely on the caregivers to do just that. Calendars provide everyone involved in the care process with a structure to follow and abide by.

IN A COMMUNITY SETTING

I had been working at the assisted living community for nearly six months, and I was starting to notice an interesting pattern with the residents. One of the first things that I had done upon starting there was to create a calendar. This calendar offered slightly different activities each day but always at the same times and in the same rooms. After a few months of using this calendar daily, I began to notice that my residents would slowly congregate in the area where the next activity was happening. One of my residents, Lucille, sat on the couch. "Hey!" she called to me when I walked in the room. "What's happening in here next?" I was surprised, as Lucille did not often seem interested in activities. "How'd you know we were getting ready to do something?" I asked her, curious. She shrugged. "I don't know, this just seemed like the place where something was supposed to happen next." Lucille had moved from one living room space to another down the hall, just because she felt like something was supposed to be going on in that new space—and she was right.

Most people associate dementia with memory problems. And while it is true that short-term memory is often impaired, people living with dementia can still learn new habits and routines. You will find that residents in care community settings always gravitate toward the same dining room chairs, the same couches, the same bedrooms. I have seen a lot of bickering break out over misplaced chairs and other furniture. Once, in the first community where I worked, I moved a piano from one side of the room to the other. My residents spent nearly a whole week complaining to me about how much they hated where the piano had been moved to. The group of ladies couldn't remember what they had had for breakfast, but they were fixated on the sudden movement of this piano from one corner to another. "Move that piano back to where it was," they'd say to me every morning. "We hate it in this new spot!" I nearly moved the piano back, but by the end of the week they'd forgotten about it.

Calendars are important in care communities. A good calendar is varied, offers different activities for different types of residents, and provides time for entertainment and outings. Here is an example layout of a strong, dementia-friendly calendar:

8 am   Breakfast

9 am   Newspapers given to those who like them

10 am   Morning physical exercise warm-up and stretching
            as a group

10:30 am	Snack break—snack cart comes around to everyone in the community
11 am	Arts and crafts or an outing, such as a lunch outing to a nearby restaurant
12 pm	Lunch
1 pm	Entertainment comes into the community or sing-along is hosted
2 pm	Small group activities led by care staff, such as folding towels or sorting socks
2:30 pm	Snack break
3 pm	Exercise program such as seated soccer or balloon toss
4 pm	Individualized activities such as nail painting led by care staff
5 pm	Dinner
6:30 pm	Small group activities like towel folding and sock sorting led by care staff
7:00 pm	Final snack before bed

If you are in charge of creating your community's calendar, you have a wide range of options and activities to choose from. You will need to work around your care community's meals and regular schedule, but this calendar allows for a lot of flexibility. Set goals for yourself each day: try to include an arts and crafts project, an outing or entertainment, physical exercise, music, small group activities like folding or sorting, and individualized activities, like nail painting or hand massages. Your goal should be to include as many varied activities as possible but always in the same physical spaces and around the same time. What you will find is that your residents start going to the same physical spaces around the same time each day. For example, if you always host crafts in the activity room, residents will start venturing there before you even begin the craft. Take advantage of your residents' patterns and natural internal clocks to make daily planning easier.

The reason that you want to include an outing earlier in the day is because it can help with sundowning in the afternoon. Sundowning— a syndrome associated with dementia where a person becomes more agitated in the afternoons and evenings—is most likely to occur when people have slept too much during the day and have been largely inactive. You want to include exercise in the afternoon for the same reason: you want your residents to get physical exercise, get their blood flowing, and keep them awake for longer and later in the day.

Notice that this calendar has three snack times, each one scheduled for about two hours after a meal. People living with dementia will not often ask for a snack or a drink of water, and they may even forget that they haven't eaten for a while, but they will happily accept these things if they are handed to them. Great snack carts have options on them for people with different dietary needs: pudding for people on puree diets and cheese and crackers for residents on regular diets, for example. Many people with dementia do not drink enough fluids, and so they are at risk for dehydration. The snack cart also helps head off this problem, as it provides both snacks and drinks.

Getting the Staff Involved

The best thing that you can do as the person in charge of the calendar is to get the rest of the staff involved in activities and resident engagement. This is always a challenging task, as many staff members respond by saying they don't have time or that it's not their job. However, there is plenty of time to put a box of socks or towels on a table and plenty of time to gather a small group of residents to work on that project. The care that hands-on staff members provide residents should be holistic, and that includes getting residents to participate in activities and to engage. There are a number of spaces in the calendar example that save room for hands-on care staff to set up activities. What often works best is to assign certain care staff members to certain activity times each morning. At 2:00 pm, for example, Vanessa is in charge of leading the activities. She has a goal of getting eight residents involved in various hands-on activities, and all of the hands-on activities are organized into boxes in a nearby cabinet. Here are some examples of activity boxes that should be available, clean, and organized every day for care staff to utilize:

- Sock sorting box: Baby socks work best because they are cute and do not end up on residents' feet. Purchase numerous colors and patterns for residents to gush over while they are sorting them.

- Towel folding box: Small, inexpensive hand towels can be found at any dollar store.

- Flower arranging box: Fake flowers and plastic vases are great ways for residents to get creative and hands on.

- Tupperware and matching lids: Everyone has spent time organizing their plastic ware cabinets, and asking residents to help you match up lids to containers is a great activity.

- Big puzzles: Puzzles that are not childish but also easy to see and hold are perfect. Puzzles should have fewer than fifty pieces.

- Silverware sorting box: Residents can help you organize your silverware drawer.

Vanessa should start the session with her residents by asking them to "help her" with any of these activities she lays out. Care staff members know the residents better than anyone else in the community, and often they know best what their residents like and don't like. While care staff may push back at first, saying, "I don't know how," or, "There's no time," they often come to find that getting residents engaged is much easier than they anticipated. When residents are engaged in an activity, they are also less likely to be falling, getting in fights with each other, or asking to use the bathroom. Care staff members come to find that taking ten minutes to set up their residents with a simple activity actually saves them time later in the day. It helps if the whole staff, from the marketing department to the housekeeper, is on board with the type of engagement and care being provided for the residents. When care staff accept from the beginning that part of their daily duties is to help with activities, they are much more likely to feel like these tasks are important and not to be neglected.

It is also important to block out time in the activity calendar for the lead activity director to plan and prepare for the next activity. When care staff are involved in activity engagement, it takes pressure off of activity directors. They are able to sit down and plan the next month's calendar or follow up on paperwork. Activity directors should strive to spend about 90 percent of their day with the residents.

AT HOME

Just because your loved one lives at home does not mean that they shouldn't have a calendar and pattern for their days. So many family caregivers have told me that their loved one doesn't like to do anything except watch TV, for example. People living with dementia will watch TV and sleep all day if you do not provide other options. Asking someone with dementia what they want to do for the day is too open ended to allow for an answer. Most people living with dementia will just say they don't know or that they don't want to do anything because there are either too many options or not enough options to choose from. Dementia prevents people from making plans, executing plans, or creating an interesting day for themselves. Some people living with dementia are also too embarrassed to attempt anything during the day. They don't want to fail or feel silly, so they will choose to do something easy, like watching TV.

People with a cognitive disease rely on their caregivers for choices and daily engagement. They need the help of their caregivers, as daunting a task as that may be, to be productive and active throughout the day. Without that assistance, people living with dementia will not make decisions and will therefore end up doing nothing. The approach that caregivers should take is to ask their loved ones with dementia whether they can help them with this or that task. This strategy allows caregivers to make their loved ones feel useful and important. Even a simple question like "Can you help me on this trip to the grocery store?" is likely to get a positive response. This question is different from "Do you want to go to the grocery store?" or "Do you want to help me?" "Can you help me" implies that you need help, not that you are necessarily asking for it. Caregivers will also benefit from offering two options to their loved ones with dementia. "Do you want eggs or pancakes for breakfast?" is a much easier question to answer than "What do you want for breakfast?" Fixed-choice questions are infinitely easier for people with dementia to answer than open-ended ones.

Making a calendar for home can be easy, stress-free, and even fun. The calendar allows caregivers and people with dementia to stick to a plan. It may also give the person with dementia a sense of normalcy: they are presented with a daily task sheet, and they know they need to do the things on this sheet. Providing two options for each activity is a great way to help people with dementia feel autonomous. They are able to choose rather than being told what exactly is happening each day. Here is an example of a great in-home calendar:

8 am	Breakfast options: eggs and toast or pancakes
9:30 am	Daily indoor stretch or walk around the neighborhood
11 am	Soap operas on TV or prelunch nap
12 pm	Lunch options: grilled cheese or turkey sandwich
1 pm	Outing or arts and crafts

3 pm	Help with chores: fold towels or dust surfaces
4 pm	Soap operas on TV or predinner nap
5 pm	Dinner options: lasagna or caesar salad
6 pm	Evening physical stretch or musical engagement

Of course, you would adjust this to meet your own schedule, but these options offer a hypothetical structure for the day. I often meet caregivers who say, "I just don't know what to do with my mom all day." If you have a calendar laid out ahead of time, you will never be at a loss for something interesting to do.

I recommend having organized boxes of activities that are ready to go. A quick trip to the dollar store can provide you with colorful socks for sorting, hand towels for folding, artificial flowers for arranging, and any number of other items that can be used for hands-on, easy activities. What you are doing with this calendar is not only offering choices to your loved one with dementia but also a structure that you can rely on.

Provide time in the calendar for you to get things done. While your loved one is watching soap operas or folding towels, you can be in another space of the house, working on something else. I always recommend, of course, that you not be the only caregiver for your loved one with dementia. Hiring someone from a home care agency or bringing in another paid caregiver is a great way to give yourself a much-needed break. Even with an outside caregiver in place, however, you are still going to want a calendar for them to follow.

Keep in mind that following a calendar of activities may also help prevent sundowning in loved ones with dementia living at home. In addition to organizing exercise routines and activities, other ways to minimize the risk is to help your loved one to avoid large meals as well as caffeine and alcohol. And you may even want to look into turning up the lights in your home when the person with dementia gets agitated or confused. Using a full-spectrum fluorescent light and placing it near your loved one for a couple of hours in the morning has also shown promise in ameliorating the change in circadian rhythms (the sleep-wake cycle) that occurs with sundowning (Khachiyants, Trinkle, Son, & Kim, 2011). Everything suggests that developing a predictable routine is most important, and having a calendar ensures that this is more likely to occur.

You will come to find that your loved one's sleep cycle and patterns begin to adhere to the schedule over time. Even if they cannot look at the calendar and make a decision by themselves, you will find that they sit down at the dining room table around lunchtime, head to the living room for activities later in the day, and even sit down in a comfy chair for a nap at the right moment. Take advantage of what you already know about your loved one's habits and sleep cycle, and then plan around that. Try to avoid forcing your loved one into habits that don't come naturally. For example, if your loved one likes to nap at 3 pm, let them nap at 3 pm. Work with that internal clock instead of against it, and you will find that you have a much easier day.

5

Embracing the Reality of People Living with Dementia

When I first started working in dementia caregiving, I learned that we should "never lie" to a person living with dementia. After only a few months of working in the field, however, I came to realize that this theory of communication was incomplete. Instead, we need to learn how to Embrace Their Reality in dementia care. What it means to embrace someone's reality is that you accept that that person no longer necessarily lives in the same world as you do. For example, if your loved one says things like "I saw my mother yesterday," even though their mother has been dead for years, instead of correcting your loved one, you say "That's great. What did you all talk about?"

Jumping into your loved one's reality takes practice. Many family members have said to me that they feel like they are lying when they embrace their loved ones' reality.

"I don't want to lie to my mom," Kara said, sighing. "But she just keeps asking where Dad is . . . so I tell her the truth. I tell her that he's dead," she explained. "Sometimes, Mom gets upset. She'll say things like, 'You never told me he died,' but then sometimes she'll remember. She will say, 'Oh, yes, I forgot that he died.' I don't know what to do."

What I recommended Kara do was this: ask her mom where she thought her husband was and then agree with her answer. "Where's your father?" Hillary asked her daughter. "Where do you think he is?" Kara responded. "Hmm . . . ," Hillary thought. "He's probably at work," she said. Instead of arguing, Kara agreed. "He's probably at work," she said back. An hour later, Kara's mother asked about him again. This time, Kara had an answer prepared. "I think you told me that he's at work," Kara said. "Oh, yes, he must be at work," her mother replied, smiling, and went back to watching TV.

Kara let her mother guide *her* into an answer. She did not have to be creative, make something up, or get into an argument about where her dad was. Instead, she responded to Hillary's question with another question. When you know what their answer is to a question like this, then you can reuse it later. Phrasing it like "I think you told me . . ." makes many family members feel better. They do not feel as though they are lying because they are only agreeing with what they have already heard.

In the past, health care practitioners were taught to correct people with dementia. This was called "reorienting" people to our reality. So, in the case of Kara and Hillary, instead of Kara agreeing that her father was at work, she would actually say something like "Mom, if you remember correctly, he died years ago." I still encounter these practices on a regular basis: explaining my concept of Embracing Their Reality is the most challenging part of working in dementia care.

When you work hands on with people living with dementia, you quickly realize that arguing and trying to correct them does not go well. In fact, it usually just ends in both parties feeling angry and frustrated. Embracing someone's reality is, by contrast, to adopt a person-centered approach to care, one that takes the best interests of the individual into consideration.

The agitation and frustration associated with the cognitive declines in persons with dementia are often ameliorated with this approach. This is why, in my work, I often encourage caregivers to throw the word "lying" out: when it's true for the person living with dementia, it's true for us, as well. When we get caught up with this word, embracing the reality of someone with dementia becomes challenging. Dementia caregiving is very much a gray area: your loved one's cognitive state ebbs and flows, and your approach needs to adjust in light of these changes. This is why it is much easier to let your loved one guide you into their world—it becomes your job just to follow, and not to correct.

IN A COMMUNITY SETTING

Dave was sure that his wife's room was right next door to his. Unfortunately for him, this was not the case. However, the thin, blonde resident next door, did, in a way, resemble his late wife. The staff at the community was less than thrilled with Dave's adoration for his neighbor and usually tried to correct him. "Dave, that's not your wife," they'd argue. "Patty has been dead for years." Dave, always in good spirits, seemed not to hear or understand them. He spent many of his days walking down the hall hand-in-hand with "Patty." Conveniently for Dave, "Patty" was also quite sure that they were married.

Dementia care communities are built for—or should be built for—the purpose of embracing the realities of their residents. Care staff must be trained and educated in order for them to be able to embrace residents' realities, which means no arguing, no disagreeing, and no reorienting residents to our world.

This also means that communities should physically and environmentally embrace the realities of their residents. For example, an "orientation board" is an unnecessary—and sometimes cruel—addition to a care community. Boards that state the year, day of the week, and season can be really confusing for people who wake up thinking it is 1954. Not only can they be confusing, but they also often look childish, as if they belong in a preschool, not an aging care community. In all truth, many residents with dementia do not even read the orientation boards or retain the information they contain if they do. What is the point of telling someone that it is not the year that they think it is?

In the chapter on environmental changes, I suggest that the physical space of dementia care communities should feel different from that of other types of senior living communities. People with dementia deserve a physical space that embraces their reality. My favorite example of a dementia care community that does embrace the reality of its residents is Hogewey in the Netherlands (dementiavillage.com/en). It is a community that is built like a small town, but it is a small town that houses only people with dementia. The care staff that work there also "work" in the little town shops: the post office, the grocery store. Residents of Hogewey can go about their lives, living much as they always have, but within the safe borders of a community that understands and meets their needs. The physical space embraces their reality, and then the staff emotionally and verbally embrace their realities as well. By "working" in the town's stores, the caregiving staff are able to provide a watchful eye and hands-on care for their residents, all while helping them maintain their independence.

When we train direct care staff in senior living communities, we need to train them to understand and work with people who have dementia, and training them to occupy the reality of residents with dementia is imperative. And as with most strategies, it is a good idea to talk with the family about the use of this approach and the benefits to their loved one with dementia.

AT HOME

Embracing your loved one's reality at home works the same way. It is important to understand that while their physical environment may not have changed, the way they perceive it may have. I have had many family caregivers complain to me that their loved one always talks about going home when they are already home. To them, however, the physical space is not recognizable as home any longer. Family members, in particular, often have a hard time understanding this.

I often go to a client's house and find that their loved ones have hung up notes, lists, and instructions everywhere for the person with dementia to read. Instead of battling back against dementia, it is easiest when caregivers embrace their loved ones' changing brain. Recognizing that reminders and quizzing won't help is the first step to embracing someone else's reality. Recall that embracing someone's reality means that you get into their world rather than trying to pull them into ours.

For people with dementia who live at home (and, often, with their caregivers) this can be a real struggle. Family caregivers have to hear the same questions day in and day out and deal with the ups and downs of twenty-four seven dementia caregiving. I often recommend that families who insist on keeping a loved one at home look into respite care, adult day care, or hiring a home care agency. It's impossible to take care of someone with dementia all day, every day, and still maintain your own peace and sanity. It is healthiest for both parties to have some time apart, and I have found that the happiest caregivers are ones that utilize respite options. It is a lot easier to embrace the reality of a loved one with dementia when you are able to take some time away from them.

Autobiographical Memory as a Tool in Dementia Care Activities

Planning a great calendar, starting great activities, and getting people engaged and excited all start with the understanding that dementia impairs a lot of different brain functions. Most notably, of course, many causes of dementia affect the short-term memory abilities of people living with dementia. Knowing this, we need to focus on using long-term memories as a way to connect with people living with dementia.

SHORT-TERM MEMORY

The first thing to go, in a lot of different types of dementia, is a person's short-term memory. For many people, this is also the first thing that presents a real challenge. What did I have for breakfast? When is that doctor's appointment? Why am I getting lost in this familiar spot? What's that word I am looking for? These and other questions often present themselves this way to a person even in early stages of dementia. From things that happened five minutes ago to events that occurred a week ago or more, many people with dementia have trouble recalling short-term memories. Caregivers can become frustrated when their loved ones repeat questions that they asked only a few minutes before. "Mom, you just asked me that, and I already told you the answer!" is something I've overheard a number of caregivers telling their loved ones with dementia. It's hard for care partners to understand that their relatives or friends are not asking questions again and again to be annoying but because they do not recall that they've already asked. Knowing this, we as caregivers need to rely on what people with dementia do have and retain throughout most of the disease process: their long-term memory.

Long-term memory is memory that has been crystalized over time. Long-term autobiographical memories are those things that are emotionally salient to the person (Conway & Pleydell-Pearce, 2000). Memories such as the birth of a child, a wedding, or a death of a close friend or family member tend to stick around. Other long-term memories, such as growing up in a certain home, the joy of riding bikes with the neighborhood kids, or where someone went to school also tend to be recalled.

While some minor changes and even losses in memory functions are to be expected as we age, the type of loss seen in dementia is not normal. We have all walked into a room and forgotten why we went in there in the first place. When "normal" forgetfulness begins to impact daily life in a routine and disabling way, however, that is when dementia may be a concern.

TIMELINE CONFUSION

"I was spending time with my mother the other day. She has advanced dementia, but she's always really pleasant. I realized, though, that she is not always sure why I call her 'Mom.' The other day she said to me, 'You know, I recognize you, but I am not quite sure who you are.' What I have come to realize is that she always loves me, and knows that she knows me, even if she can't figure out who I am that day," Sally told me, smiling.

In my experience, time is not linear for people living with dementia. They will talk about things like where they grew up, or what their parents are doing, as if these things are happening presently. Often, long-term memories become intermingled with short-term past memories or worries and concerns about the future. You may hear someone with dementia talk about their parents picking them up after school in one sentence and then, a second later, make a reference to watching their first child get married. I call this concept Timeline Confusion. People living with dementia often have a very hard time understanding the concept of time. This is why people with dementia will occasionally have trouble recognizing their loved ones. It is not that they do not know them; rather they cannot place them on a timeline that makes sense. For example, if your mother believes that it is 1970 and that you are 15, she may have trouble "placing" you when you visit with her. She is looking for a 15-year-old, and you aren't 15, so she chooses the next best option: you're her friend, neighbor, maybe even her sister. Your mother knows that she knows you, but she cannot place you on a timeline that makes sense to her.

UNDERSTANDING

Chrissy seemed to be doing well enough. The home care agency I worked with had sent me to assess her, knowing that she had some dementia. I was curious, based on what I had read about her, if I would see much of her impairment. For the most part, Chrissy was very "with it." She was well-spoken and witty, and even her short-term memory did not seem to be too poor. As we sat at her kitchen counter talking, I watched for signs of her impairment.

"If you'll excuse me, I'd like to make a phone call," she said. "Oh, of course," I nodded. Chrissy reached for her TV remote and looked at it. I saw her brow furrow as she tried to figure out what to do next.

Chrissy began dialing numbers into the TV remote, pressing each key slowly. "I'm trying . . . to remember what . . . his number is," she offered as a reason for her struggle. I reached across the counter and got her phone. "Let's try this, instead," I said. Not wanting to embarrass her, I added, "Sometimes the remote and the phone look similar!" "Oh, right, yes . . ." Chrissy trailed off, dialing the number into her phone.

Not only is memory affected by dementia but a person's ability to conceptualize and understand is also jeopardized. I didn't want to embarrass Chrissy, so I cautiously slipped the phone in front of her. If it was not for me, however, I do not believe that Chrissy would have realized she was making a mistake by dialing into the remote. This act alone made me much more confident of her impairment than anything else she did or said during our time together.

Imagine information processing in dementia to be like a large, five-hundred-piece puzzle. If you took that puzzle and dumped all of the pieces all over the table, you would have quite a mess. Technically, you could make any of those pieces fit together if you wanted them to. You could pick up two pieces and shape them and with the help of some tape and scissors make a fit. Now, these pieces wouldn't actually fit or make sense together, but you can imagine that this is what it is like for people with dementia: they find themselves putting together a lot of ill-fitting puzzle pieces. People with dementia will frequently take pieces of information that they have heard or seen and put it together with other pieces of information that they've heard or seen. What you end up with is a lot of confusion and not a lot of logic. This is also why utilizing logic to argue with or convince someone with dementia doesn't typically work: their logic is inherently flawed. When people living with dementia become confused, they reinvent their world so that they can accommodate their new logic. Chrissy's excuse for using the TV remote as a phone was that she was "too busy focusing on remembering the right phone number," which obviously would not impair most people to the point that they would use a TV remote to make a phone call. However, due to Chrissy's confusion, even her excuse had to fit in with the rest of her logic. To be clear, Chrissy did not cover for her mistakes on purpose: her brain just found ways to make sense of what was confusing to her.

PERCEPTION

The way a person with dementia perceives the world around them also changes. For example, I have watched residents with dementia lean down to the carpet to try to pull patterns off the floor. If a carpet has thick lines on it, sometimes they will spend time trying to pick up the lines. If a fabric chair has a leaf pattern, sometimes they will try and pick up the leaves. To the person with dementia, the lines on the carpet and the leaves on the chair look and feel like they are three dimensional even though they're not. People with dementia have trouble with perception in both a physical and emotional sense. If something looks and feels real, a person with dementia may perceive it as real.

UTILIZING THIS KNOWLEDGE

Knowing all of this is the first step in making a dementia care environment happy for someone with dementia. Now that we understand how short-term memory, understanding, and perception change in dementia, we need to incorporate these items into our activity and engagement calendar. We need to plan activities that make sense for people with these types of impairments. When I make recommendations to new activity directors (or family caregivers, for that matter), I always encourage them to utilize the long-term memory of people who are living with dementia. Since long-term memory stays intact longer, offering activities that rely on long-term memory is the best thing that you can do.

Here are some examples of using long-term memory, understanding, and perception in daily activities, and why each works or does not work.

PHOTO ALBUMS

I have been to many, many dementia care workshops and heard many different people speak about dementia care. At nearly every event I attend, someone recommends using photo albums with people who have dementia. While I think that this can be a good activity, I believe the idea of incorporating photo albums started because caregivers thought it would help their loved ones "remember." This is where I caution caregivers: do not use photo albums for the purpose of "jogging" someone's memory. Photo albums can prompt long-term memory, but many people with dementia will recall information incorrectly. It's important for caregivers not to correct their loved ones with dementia even when they get identities wrong. For example, if a woman with dementia believes that the little boy in the photo is her son rather than her brother, that is okay. Correcting her will only bring more confusion and frustration. Photo albums can be really enjoyable for caregivers and people with dementia alike, but we want to be sure not to use them for recall purposes.

A resident I worked with was visited by her family. She smiled at each of her family members but didn't say anything, despite their many attempts to engage her in simple conversation. One of her sons took a photo off the wall of about fifteen families that she had spent time with as an overseas missionary and asked his mom if she remembered any of those people. Her face lit up as she accurately named every adult and child in the photo!

I share this because sometimes photos can be good ways to tap those long-term memories, but it may not work for everyone. It is important to let the person with dementia respond in their own way. With this example, if the individual simply smiled as she looked at the photo, that might have been enough. If she was not interested and looked away, that would be acceptable as well.

BABY DOLLS AND STUFFED ANIMALS

Knowing what we know about perception and understanding in dementia, it makes sense that impaired individuals will often believe baby dolls and stuffed animals are real. If they look real enough and feel real enough, they are often real to the person with dementia. These products can be wonderful tools. I caution, though, against using teddy bears or unrealistic stuffed animals or dolls. These can be confusing. No one keeps a real bear in their house, and certainly not a small bear with a red bow tie. Use products that are dignified and realistic when working with people who have dementia. I discuss this in much more depth and breadth in chapter 11.

7

Group Dynamics

This chapter is written primarily for people who work in dementia care communities or adult day care communities and describes ways to communicate and engage with older adults with dementia in group or individual settings.

Amanda was one of my favorite people. She was in an advanced stage of dementia but very pleasant and friendly. Amanda had aphasia, which meant that she had trouble communicating verbally. Despite this difficulty with verbal communication, Amanda was very expressive. She would actually mime laughing or talking and would often grab my hand when she heard music, turning me around to dance with her.

Although she was one of my favorite residents to spend time with, Amanda was particularly disruptive in group settings. She would often annoy the other residents by commandeering an entertainer's attention, getting up to shake her bum for the piano player who came to visit once a month, for example. "Sit down! You're embarrassing yourself!" other ladies would yell at her.

Amanda thought of this behavior as comical—which, in a way, it was—but my other residents did not enjoy it. Because her memory was so poor, we could not tell her that she'd already done this "joke" three times and that people were getting upset. Often, I would get another staff member to engage with Amanda when I started a group activity during which she might become disruptive.

LARGE GROUPS

One of the most frequent complaints I hear from activity directors is that they can't get any of their residents to sit down and stay seated for an activity and that any time they go to get other residents, the ones they had already seated get up and leave. I have also heard things like "This one resident is really disruptive" and "None of my residents want to do anything, or one says no, and they all say no." These are all normal problems, and they all have easy fixes.

GETTING RESIDENTS TO SAY YES

More than once, I have had a wonderful group of residents who loved to go on outings, do crafts, and exercise together. More than once, too, I have had one of those residents become despondent and start saying no to everything that was suggested. When one of the residents that says no is an influential person, other people will often say no as well. I think of it as a "group mind" sort of influence. If one person hears another saying no, they may also say no because it feels comfortable and familiar.

Jack had some sort of magical influence with his fellow residents. He was high functioning and smart, so that may have been part of it. Whatever Jack said, went. If he didn't want to participate in an activity, no one did. If he wanted to go on an outing, everyone wanted to go. Upon being asked if she'd enjoy going out for ice cream, Rebecca asked, "Is Jack going?" The key became to get Jack to agree, and then everyone would agree.

I realized that there was a lot of power in positivity. I would often promise Jack that it would be a good time and encourage him to help us round up other people to go. Because he was quite popular, if he was inviting someone, they would often agree to come along.

It became a useful trick to get Jack to gather up some friends for a successful trip.

Many people living with dementia will default to no if they do not know what the other options are, or if they feel like whatever you are asking will be too much work, or if they don't understand what you are asking. For some residents, telling them to come with you is the best approach. I have often led residents on outings just by taking their hands and telling them that they'll have fun. Once I am able to draw someone like Jack whom the group feels is the leader into an activity, others will often follow suit.

GETTING GROUPS TO STAY PUT

When you are starting a large activity, getting your group of residents to stay seated can be a real challenge. As you drop off three residents and go to get another one from the hallway, two from the first group get bored waiting for you and leave the room. You come back with one resident in tow, but now half your group is missing. You have to start all over again.

Many people living with dementia have very short attention spans. I have found, in practice, that group activities should not go longer than forty-five minutes. After about forty-five minutes, even if the activity is fun and your residents are enjoying themselves, many of them will start to get antsy and agitated. Here are some tips to help get residents to stay for an activity that you're starting:

1. Plan ahead of time: make sure the activity will last less than an hour.

2. Choose which residents you'll be bringing to the activity before you go and get them.

3. It helps to know your residents well enough to know who will enjoy what you're starting.

4. Have another staff member help you. Ask someone to bring a few residents into the room where you're beginning the activity.

5. Start the activity as soon as the residents enter the room. For example, even if you aren't ready to put the cookies in the oven, let your first residents assemble the cooking items on the table. Get them involved in something so that they don't get bored and leave before you get back with everyone else.

6. Do not get frustrated if you lose a few people. This happens, and it is very normal. For whatever reason, some of your residents will get up and leave the activity. It is not your fault, and you know better for next time who will enjoy what you're doing.

Above all else, getting large groups of residents together for an activity takes practice. It takes knowing your residents well, and it takes some rushing around. The best activities are those that are simple, fun, and start immediately.

WORKING WITH A DISRUPTIVE RESIDENT

In the story I shared, Amanda is a perfect example of the resident who can be disruptive at times. Despite the fact that she was one of my favorite people, she was also one of the more difficult residents to work with. Even when an activity was going well, she would run into the middle of the group and frustrate the other residents. When I had a feeling that Amanda would be coming to the activity, invited or not, I employed a few simple techniques:

1. I would separate her from the group activity by asking a staff member to engage her in another room.

2. I would find a specific "job" for Amanda to do within the larger group. For example, I sometimes had her play "goalie" if the ball we were using went outside the circle the residents were kicking it back and forth within.

3. I would choose an activity that I knew would be better suited for Amanda or else one that would bore her. In either case, she would either engage appropriately or leave if it didn't suit her.

There will always be residents who make group activities more challenging. The key is to find ways to engage with them without them upsetting the rest of the group.

SMALLER GROUPS

Small groups are best if you are planning an outing or a more challenging craft activity. Within every group of residents, there tends to be a smaller group that can handle an extra-challenging event. Outings, in particular, can be difficult for some people with dementia. For example, someone who needs to constantly use the restroom will not fare well on a trip to the zoo where bathrooms tend to be few and far between. A resident who becomes frustrated quickly may not do well on an outing that requires a half-hour drive.

A tradition that the assisted living community had kept up was taking residents to the town's Christmas parade. Although I had chosen my residents carefully for this event, I made an error in judgement. Lucille and Dot were roommates, and Dot went nowhere without her companion. Lucille, however, was much harder to take on excursions, even in small groups. She got agitated quickly and did not like long bus rides. Knowing that I could not take Dot without

Lucille, I decided to take both of them. About ten minutes into the ride, however, Lucille started getting agitated. "I have to pee!" she called from her seat. "Where's the bathroom?" Even though we only had ten residents on the bus, the entire trip quickly devolved. We managed to pull over and find a restroom before the parade started, but it was not long before Lucille became agitated with the parade itself. "Why is this so long?" she cried out.

When I am planning a smaller group event, I look for residents who naturally pair off together. Although this can sometimes be a challenge, such as in the case of Lucille and Dot, friends tend to balance each other out. When one is going on an outing, I also take the other one. Creating small groups is easier than creating larger groups, but it also takes a little more planning. You want to look for residents that get along with each other or at least do not dislike each other. Despite their memory problems, I have found that people with dementia remember their "enemies," even if they met that person recently. On outings, I take only six or seven residents with dementia. More than that and groups become too large and unwieldy. A small group should really not have more than eight residents. Even when you are doing an intricate craft, more than eight people is a challenging number to handle by yourself.

ONE-ON-ONE

For some residents, one-on-one activities are best. Some people are more introverted than others, and even the smallest of groups may be a deterrent to getting involved. I have also seen situations where residents whose dementia is more advanced than in others tend to distance themselves for fear of being made fun of or ostracized. In many cases, the people who are most progressed in their dementia are isolated from others, just because of the nature of the disease. These residents will often stay in their rooms, and some are even bedbound near the end of their lives.

Every day, I had made it a point to visit Miranda in her room. She was actively hallucinating and often distracted by the "children" she saw in her room. Miranda was not stuck in bed, but she mostly sat in her lounge chair. While she physically could have come out of the room, she greatly preferred not to. "Woah, woah!" she'd cry if someone tried to wheel her outside the room in her wheelchair. "Take me back!"

I did not see the point in forcing Miranda to come out of her room when she didn't want to. Her family, on the other hand, wanted her to get the maximum amount of socialization possible. "Mom always loved groups," Miranda's daughter told me. "Bring her out when you all are doing a craft or music activity, please." I tried to explain to Miranda's daughter that her mother's needs and wants had changed with her dementia. Not only was she more comfortable if the activity came to her, but she also seemed much more engaged in a one-on-one setting.

Nearly any activity can be turned into a one-on-one program, although some work better than others. Especially when someone is on hospice and near the end of their life, activities need to be adjusted to meet their needs. One program that I always loved was a type of solace program that my senior living community offered. Staff members would take turns throughout the day visiting residents in their rooms who were on hospice. They would go in, provide individualized attention, and make sure that a music player was playing the residents' favorite tunes. Here are some examples of individualized activities that we used:

- Hand massage with a wet, warm washcloth

- Favorite music and song discussions

- Asking for help with a "chore," such as towel folding

- Fingernail painting

- Salon hair care, either having the hairstylist come to them or bringing them to the salon when no one else is there

- Looking through photo albums

- Individual entertainment, such as a guitar player coming in to sing with the resident

When making the monthly calendar, we set aside time for staff members to spend with residents one-on-one. Without the time blocked out in the calendar, we knew that when the staff got busy, the individual residents would be forgotten. For example, we set aside time at 10:30 am, 2:30 pm, and 6:30 pm, on the calendar for a staff member to visit isolated residents for just fifteen minutes apiece. While it doesn't seem like a lot of time, there are many communities that do not take the time to even offer fifteen minutes to bedbound residents. Even though they do not leave their rooms, these residents still deserve the love and attention that the other residents receive, and in ways that are most meaningful to them.

SUMMING IT UP

If you are the person who creates the monthly calendar, I recommend offering each of these three types of group activities a day. At least one or two activities should be for large groups and a few should be for smaller groups, and there also ought to be ongoing individualized activities throughout the day. While there will always be pushback from the staff, often in the form of "We don't have time," the staff's sole purpose is to care for the residents who live in the community. Making time for them, whether in groups or through individual activities, is vital.

8

Asking for Help

Eric sat in his La-Z-Boy brown leather armchair, feet propped up, head facing the TV screen. Eric, however, was hardly watching the soap opera. I was pretty sure that had someone asked him what the show was about, he would not be able to answer. His caregiver was a professional from a local nonmedical home care company. She was good at her job and took a lot of pride in making sure the house looked great and that Eric got his medicine and meals on time. Other than that, though, she was not sure how to engage this man with dementia in anything except watching television. "I've asked him what he wants to do," she assured me. "But he says he doesn't want to do anything at all, so I just let him watch TV." "That's the problem," I replied. "He doesn't know what options are available to him, so he'll just say that he doesn't want to do anything!"

Even when Eric heard his options and was asked which of the things he might like to do, he did not fully understand the question. "Do you want to go for a walk, do you want to paint this birdhouse with me inside, or do you want to watch TV?" the caregiver would ask him. Eric would just shrug and respond, "I don't know." He was being honest: he really did not know, because his dementia did not allow him to fully comprehend the question. Instead of choosing one of those confusing options, he just told his caregiver that he didn't really want to do any of them.

Everyone in the world (or most people, at least) want to feel useful, helpful, and necessary. People with dementia, however, too often get pushed to the side. "Well, Mom can't clean the counters like she used to, so I'll just do it," family members say. The same thing happens in senior living communities. "A few of our residents can't cut their own food very well, so we'll just save time and cut up everyone's food for them," staff members explain. These family and professional caregivers are not trying to take things away from people with dementia—they are just trying to make everyone's lives a little easier. What they are doing, though, is making it too easy for the person living with dementia. Now that person will rely on their caregiver for absolutely everything. Caregivers do everything from cutting up their food to changing the TV channel, and so people with dementia are given almost zero responsibility. This makes them feel useless, bored, and unnecessary—and who wants to feel that way?

How do we fix this problem? How do we make people with dementia feel useful and engaged? How do we get them to do activities, even when it seems like they don't want to do anything at all? The good news is that there is a simple fix.

ASKING FOR HELP

I often use this analogy with new caregivers. Let's pretend you have a neighbor who is moving out of one house and into another down the road. "Hey, *do you want* to help me move this weekend?" your friend asks you. Your stomach drops and you panic, pulling out your phone's calendar in the hopes that something else will be taking up your time that weekend. You don't want to help your friend move! Moving someone is a real pain. You wish he'd just hire a moving company.

Pretend next that your friend approaches you a little differently. "Hey, *can* you help me move this weekend?" he asks you. It's the same question, but it's phrased differently. He is not asking if you *want* to do something, he's asking if you *can* do something. It seems silly, but it really is a different question. You still don't want to do it, but your friend has asked for your help. He needs you. You take a deep breath and nod. "I can help you move," you say.

I stumbled on this asking for help idea when I was working with groups of residents in my first care community. I recall asking a group of residents living with dementia if they wanted to paint birdhouses with me and having all of them shake their heads no. "Nope, I'm just fine here on the couch!" one of them said, smiling. I sighed and walked away. I was new to the job, and I was having a real problem getting my residents to do anything except sit around and chat. As I was walking away, I thought about the times that I'd had success getting residents to do activities with me. I realized that I had actually asked a different question. Knowing that their memories weren't the best, I waited about five minutes, and then returned to the group. "Hey, *can* you all *help* me paint some birdhouses? I could really use some assistance getting the courtyard spruced up!" All of my residents nodded, got up, and followed me to the activity room.

It really is as simple as it seems. The question needs to be "Can you help me?" It cannot be any of the following:

- Do you want to help me?

- How about you come help me?

- Do you feel like helping me?

- Would you like to help me?

I have watched caregivers use these phrasings and then turn to me and say, "See! Asking for help doesn't work!" The problem was that the caregiver didn't ask for help but instead asked if the person wanted to, felt like, or could help them with something. "Can you" is a completely different way to phrase the question, and it means something different.

USING "HELP" IN CHORES OR ACTIVITIES

"Hey, Mom, I've got some dishes in the sink that I have to wash and dry. Can you help me with these?" Ed asked, motioning to the sink. She nodded and immediately began taking wet dishes from him and drying each one carefully. What Ed's mother didn't realize was that these were the same dishes she'd dried yesterday, the day before, and the day before that. Ed had found a great way to get his mother ready and awake for breakfast: start her on a dish-drying routine.

While almost no one likes to do chores around the house, I have found that people living with dementia actually do enjoy completing chores—if they feel as though they are being of use to someone else. Even when you do not need help with a chore, asking a person with dementia for help is a great way to make them feel important. Ed figured out that a great way to wake his mother up and get her brain working and her hands nimble was to have her do chores each morning.

Even if the chore is not done to your liking, it is important that you not undo it in front of the person with dementia. This will make them feel silly and most likely annoyed. If your aunt did not set the table properly, wait until she leaves the room, and then fix it.

USING "HELP" DURING SHOWERING, TOILETING, AND MORE

The beauty of the asking for help technique is that it can be used in all sorts of situations, not just ones related to crafts or chores. It can also be used to help people with dementia complete activities of daily living, or ADLs. ADLs are items like bathing, toileting, feeding, dressing—all the things that one needs to do regularly to live a healthy life.

Many caregivers struggle with getting their loved ones with dementia to complete their ADLs. Instead of fighting and arguing before each shower, try this instead: ask for help.

I recall giving one particularly "combative" resident a shower. The staff had told me that he was very aggressive, but what I came to realize was that he felt uncomfortable and didn't want to be touched without his consent (not surprising!) So I asked him for help. "Can you help me? Hold this washcloth and wash your face," I suggested. "I will wash your legs while you do that." I encouraged him and made him feel as though he was being helpful. He gladly took the washcloth and cleaned his face.

You can ask someone with dementia to show you where their bathroom is or to help you make them a sandwich for lunch. Suddenly, that person is in the shower. Suddenly, they are eating the sandwich they helped to make. "Help" comes in many forms, too: maybe she cannot make a sandwich without your help, but she can put mayonnaise on the bread.

CONCLUSION

Whatever the task may be, engaging someone living with dementia is much easier once they feel useful, purposeful, and necessary. No one wants to become a bump on a log. By asking someone for help, you are showing them that they are important and necessary. Not only can this get someone with dementia engaged in an activity but it can also lift their spirits. Being asked for assistance means that you are a worthwhile, useful individual. We can help people living with dementia to feel this way.

Activities of Daily Living

TAKING THINGS AWAY

Even though we do not mean to, we take things away from people with dementia: car keys, the ability to use the stovetop alone, the password for the online banking account. In many cases, it is necessary to do so. That said, we sometimes take things from people with dementia solely for the sake of ease. For example, an adult child may start setting the table for dinner, even though he had previously let his mom with dementia do it. The son means well, but he finished the task to save everyone time. The problem is this: even though his mom has dementia, she can still set the table for dinner—it may just take a little while longer, and the napkins may not be folded perfectly. Still, she can complete the task. Her son, without meaning to, has taken away part of her autonomy.

Although dinner had started, none of the residents had received knives. The ones that could still use utensils had forks and spoons in front of them, but no knives. Eighty-six-year-old Jack looked at his meal and then back at his place settings. He picked up his fork and began to cut his baked potato in half with it. "Oh, let me do that for you, Jack," one of the care aides said, taking the plate from him. She cut his potato in half with her knife and put the plate back down on the table. "There you are," she said, smiling. "We don't give anyone here knives to cut with," she explained to a new staff member. "People with dementia shouldn't have butter knives."

It would be nice if a story like this was uncommon, but it's not. Many people believe that adults with dementia are not "allowed" to use knives, even blunt tools like butter knives. They may be afraid a person living with dementia will hurt themselves with a blunt knife or that that person will attack someone. If someone was a large fall risk, there may be a reason to take sharp objects away, but butter knives? A dull object like this can't cause any more damage than a fork can.

Not only is taking away someone's ability to cut their own food (before they are unable to do so themselves) inappropriate but it can create more issues. Now a person like Jack has to come up with a new way to cut their food. Depending on his stage of dementia, Jack may not be able to identify what utensil is missing—he may just start having trouble eating.

LEARNED HELPLESSNESS

Caitlin could no longer use utensils, but she was still intent on feeding herself. In order to allow her to do that, Caitlin's daughter switched her to finger foods. This new finger food diet meant that everything on Caitlin's plate was something that she could pick up. Instead of a piece of chicken breast, it was cut-up chicken or chicken fingers. Instead of soup in a bowl with a spoon, it was soup in a mug that she could hold and sip. Without the finger food option, Caitlin's daughter would have had to feed her mother, thereby taking away one more thing that Caitlin could still do.

Psychologist Martin Seligman stumbled on his theory of learned helplessness while working on another project. Studying dogs and their response to a small electric shock, Seligman found that the dogs had learned that they could not control if or when the shock was coming

(Maier and Seligman, 1976). Instead of moving to another side of the room to avoid the shock, the dogs seemed to give up. In other words, they learned that they were helpless to control the situation at hand.

In one way or another, we often cause this reaction in people with cognitive impairments, especially those in the earlier stages of the disease. When we treat someone as though they cannot do something that they can still do, we teach them that they are helpless. Instead of giving a person with dementia extra time to set the table, we take over the task ourselves. Instead of allowing someone with dementia to feed themselves with finger food, we cut up their food and feed it to them.

Giving someone living with dementia the opportunity to feel a little frustration, work a little harder, and do something for themselves can pay off in a positive way. It is okay for a person with dementia to struggle a little bit to finish a task. We must remember that these are adults who have lived long, full lives. Suddenly, they have no chores, tasks, or anything of importance to do. The lives they once had, with busy schedules and plans, have dissolved. While people with dementia can't do everything they once did, they should be allowed to continue to do what they are able to do.

There are many research studies linking depression and dementia. In a 2017 study, Vyara Valkanova and team suggest that as many as 20 percent of the Alzheimer patients in their study and as many as 45 percent of their patients with vascular dementia had some level of depression. While depression can precede (and potentially cause) some cognitive impairment, it is noted that dementia and depression often coexist. While sheer biology has an effect on the interaction and link between depression and dementia, there is also the fact that many people with dementia become isolated from their peers. They are unable to do the things that they once loved to do. The tasks they once took pride in handling themselves, such as driving themselves to appointments or doing their own taxes, are now being completed by other people. The effect of environmental changes like these is such that it is no wonder that dementia and depression have such a high comorbidity.

CHORES ARE ACTIVITIES

While most people would not identify chores and tasks around the house as fun, they would probably deem them to be important. Each day, there are certain things that a person must do to keep their house or apartment nice and tidy. Sorting through the laundry, washing the dishes, and setting the table are all necessary tasks. We don't realize it, but we end up taking many of these tasks away from people with dementia. Even if a person with dementia may take far too long to set the table, there are plenty of positive reasons for them to continue working on completing tasks like this. It's imperative that we allow people with dementia to continue feeling useful and important.

Chores are an excellent way to make people with dementia feel as though their presence is necessary (figure 9.1). You can use the technique of asking for help that I describe in chapter 8 when trying to engage a person with dementia in chores. Here is a great list of chores that people with dementia can still do:

- Folding and sorting socks

- Setting the table

- Sweeping the floor

- Wiping down counters

- Washing and drying dishes

- Organizing silverware

- Folding towels

- Matching lids to containers

- Wiping down windows

- Organizing items from a desk drawer

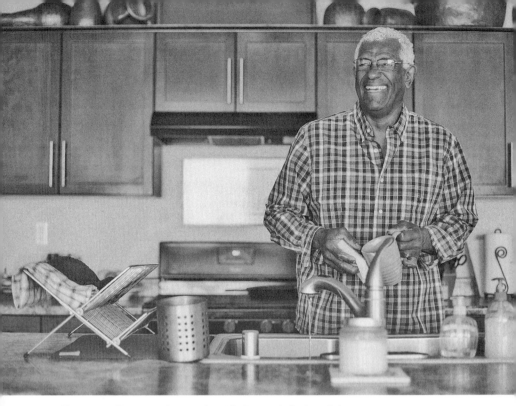

Figure 9.1. Chores make people with dementia feel useful

The great thing about all of these jobs is that they need to be done frequently. And even if you do not need help with sorting and matching socks at that given moment, there is no reason that you cannot keep a basket set aside with socks for sorting.

Tim was highly agitated and focused on leaving his house. He wanted to go pick up his daughter from the airport because he believed that she needed a ride. Tim's daughter was safe at home, but for one reason or another, this was Tim's ongoing delusion. His caregivers had a really difficult time keeping Tim relaxed and safe when he got focused on his airport plan. I taught his caregivers to utilize asking him to undertake chores around the house as a method for turning his attention to something else. Tim was chairbound for the most part, so we brought the kitchen hand towels to him. "Hey, Tim," his caregivers would say, "can you help me fold these towels? I have so much to do today!" Because Tim's dementia was so advanced, in order for him to fold the towels well, he needed to be 100 percent focused on the task. This was good news because it took Tim's attention off of the airport delusion.

Notice that we also only gave Tim one direction. People with dementia struggle when we give them multiple tasks to complete or ask them to complete a task with multiple steps (e.g., "please fold the dark towels first and then the light ones, and then put all the kitchen towels over here," etc.). Keep it to one routine task.

No matter what the chore is, it is the *doing* of it that matters, not the actual outcome. For example, although Tim was folding towels successfully, we quietly unfolded each one that he completed. In order to keep the task going and to keep Tim engaged longer, we focused on the "doing" part of the task. It did not matter how well or how poorly the towel was actually folded. One of the reasons that people with dementia stop doing tasks is because their caregivers will suggest that they can't do it well anymore. It does not really matter how well the task is done as long as the person with dementia is feeling successful doing it.

THE SMALL STUFF MATTERS

When engaging people with dementia, the small stuff matters. The things that we take for granted, like our ability to complete chores or run errands, are things a person with dementia comes to miss. No longer is it easy to carry out these tasks: now, instead of Tim worrying about ten things at once *while* folding towels, he can only fold towels. In order to get people living with dementia to feel helpful, useful, and engaged, we need to focus on the little things. Instead of taking items away (such as butter knives) we should focus on what people with dementia can still do and allow them to do it.

Tailored Activities

Molly had been a registered nurse her whole life. She'd spent the great majority of that nursing career working in senior living. Now, in an ironic twist of fate, Molly was living in a dementia care community. The good thing was this: Molly did not feel like she was living in a care community setting; in fact, she believed that she was still going to work each day.

This retired nurse could not ambulate on her own, so she spent most of her day in a high-back wheelchair. Molly often wore her glasses down the front of her nose, seemingly as part of a habit of peering at notes or patients. I'd given Molly a stethoscope and a notepad so that she could continue "working" throughout the day. Once, a resident across the dining room coughed loudly. Molly, normally an incredibly soft-spoken woman, yelled out, "Is someone planning to attend to that patient!"

People living with dementia are often left to their own devices even though we know their ability to plan (an executive function associated with the prefrontal cortex of the brain) is impacted by dementia. Further, even when options are offered, they are not as varied as may be needed. Not everyone living with dementia wants to do arts and crafts, bingo, sing, listen to music, or do physical exercise. Molly, my favorite retired nurse, was not able to do very much that involved coordination because of her Parkinson disease. Even feeding herself was a challenge. While she enjoyed singing quietly along with music, Molly's favorite activity was nursing. She had been a nurse her whole life and that was what she loved doing. Now, with dementia, Molly believed that she was still working as a nurse and supporting her in that belief gave her a way to engage that she found satisfying.

In order to find the activities that work best for people with cognitive impairments, you need to know your loved ones, your clients, your patients, your residents well enough as people to know what they like. Not everyone is going to enjoy doing bingo every day (although I have met people who do). Tailoring activities to meet the needs and interests of different people starts with an understanding of whom you are working with. Often, knowing someone's past interests, hobbies, or career is a great jumping-off point.

Too often, people with dementia who live at home end up sitting in front of the television all day. "That's what he likes to do," caregivers will say, motioning to the chair where their father spends twelve hours of his day. People living with dementia will sleep all day if you let them, and they will watch TV all day if you let them. This is not because they enjoy these things; it is just because they don't realize that there are other options. Asking someone with dementia what they want to do that day is just too complicated of a question. The list of things that that person wants to do is probably full of items that they cannot do anymore, such as drive a car, pick up their kids from school, go to work, or go on a dream vacation unattended. Being asked what they want to do is likely to remind any number of people with dementia that they cannot do much of anything without assistance anymore.

For many people, holding down a job and providing for their family were the most important things that they ever did. I recall one resident I had, Linda, who was a master's-level-educated teacher. Linda was always active and engaged in life, volunteering on numerous boards and with many clubs even after she retired. As her Alzheimer disease progressed, however, Linda could no longer do what she used to do. When she arrived at our care community at a moderate stage of dementia, Linda was newly unaware of her Alzheimer's. This was a good thing, since Linda was back to believing she was a capable, busy woman with many tasks to do. It was hard to get Linda involved in any activities, mostly because she was always "going somewhere." I would ask her, "Linda, we are getting ready for lunch, can you help me set the tables?" She'd smile, politely, and sigh. "Oh, honey, I'd love to help you, but I have a job interview coming up, and I've got to get going!" she'd say, giving me a wave and rushing off down the hallway to an interview that was never coming.

Linda was the kind of person that did not like to do the more typical activities offered in dementia care communities. Instead, Linda wanted to go to work. A lot of the staff would say that she didn't like to do anything, but that really was not the case. In fact, Linda enjoyed doing a great many things: working, volunteering, riding her bike, going on picnics, and attending parties. Sadly, Linda could not do any of these things anymore, at least not in the way that she used to do them. I was inspired by Linda and some of our other retired teachers, however, and decided to add something new to the calendar: reading to children. I found a local preschool and talked to the teachers there. Every other Tuesday, I would get my retired teachers together and get on the bus. We would go to that local preschool, and my residents with moderate to advanced dementia would open up books and read to the children. Linda absolutely loved this more unconventional activity and regularly took over the classroom duties. "Can she stay here and help us?" one of the classroom teachers asked me once.

Use people's careers as jumping-off points for activity ideas. If you are the caregiver for a relative or friend, you probably already know what they enjoy doing. In my case, collecting information from my residents' family members was crucial. Every time that we got a new resident, I would review their paperwork. I would look to see what they enjoyed, what they disliked, and what they did for a living. What follows are some great questions that you can use when trying to choose activities for people with dementia.

What did they do for a living? What a person did for a living can tell you a lot about them. A career nurse like Molly who would have worked third shift—even if it was thirty years ago—may go back to having third-shift sleeping habits. Someone who had a high-stress job may spend a lot of time acting stressed, even if there is nothing in their environment to stress about.

Where did they grow up? Knowing where someone grew up can also tell you a lot about that person. Did they grow up on a farm where they spent days being busy and active? Did they grow up in an upper-middle-class suburb where they weren't expected to do much household work? I once had a resident who refused to fold towels or sort socks because she had grown up with housekeepers who did that sort of thing for her. Household chores were never something that she had done or considered doing.

What hobbies do they have? This is one of my favorite questions to ask my new residents. There is so much that you can learn about who a person is through their hobbies. And while career paths often change, people's hobbies typically do not. Groups they volunteered with, exercise routines, and weekend activities tend to stick with people through dementia. The key here is not to ask what the person with dementia wants to do but rather what they liked to do in their free time. People with dementia will commonly say that they don't like to do anything or can't do what they used to do instead of just telling you what they actually enjoy. I have found that when people with dementia say no or decline to do things, it is not out of dislike but rather out of anxiety or fear. They are worried that they won't be able to complete a task like they used to.

Are they an introvert or an extrovert? I consider myself an extreme extrovert, and I love being around other people. Many of my activities, such as improv comedy, involve me performing or entertaining others. Knowing this about me, you would probably want to invite me to activities that a lot of other people were taking part in. I would not fare too well participating in a solitary craft or game. For me, sitting by myself for more than a couple hours is excruciating. For people who are introverts, however, tailoring their activities to include quiet or down time is important.

What types of activities or entertainment do they dislike? Knowing what someone doesn't like is almost as important as knowing what they do like. I have had residents walk out of performances by accordion players because they hate accordion music. It is particularly challenging with people who have dementia, since you cannot always predict how they are going to act or respond. I have had a number of embarrassing situations where I've invited a performer to entertain a group of residents with dementia only to have nearly everyone leave the room because I got the wrong type of entertainer. Because many people with dementia lack a filter, they will make it clear when they do not like or enjoy something that is going on.

Did they raise children, have pets, or both? I recall a day in my first job when I wanted to bring residents to a local animal shelter to pet the dogs and cats. It was a great idea in theory, but I clearly had not looked through everyone's paperwork before getting residents onto the bus. I told everyone where we were going and what we were doing, but, of course, not everyone was able to voice their opinion of the outing. I overestimated everyone's excitement in meeting dogs and cats, and Shelly was one of the first to panic. We got into the room at the animal shelter where they'd be bringing dogs and cats in. A volunteer brought in a dog, and Shelly had a complete meltdown. "Get that out of here!" she yelled, trying to kick at the dog under the table. I had to walk Shelly out of the room and apologize to the volunteer (and the dog, who was untouched and seemingly unfazed, thankfully).

Shelly, however, loved children. Whenever we visited a local preschool or had children come in to see our residents, Shelly was overjoyed—she just hated animals. If I had read her paperwork a little beforehand (or had asked her family members the right questions), we could have avoided the entire animal shelter mishap.

This is also a good question to know the answer to when trying out stuffed animals or baby dolls for people with dementia. Just as Shelly did not like real dogs, she was not interested in stuffed ones either. Because they all seemed real to her, Shelly panicked around stuffed animals as well as live ones.

Where and when do they believe that they are, currently? I have had countless caregivers state that the people they are caring for just don't like to do anything they used to like doing. I often find that this is because they were never given an option to continue doing what they enjoyed. I had one resident, Mary Ellen, who had been an artist her whole life. The entire activity staff told me when I came onboard that Mary Ellen didn't like to paint anymore. I decided to test out that theory and set out some paints and canvas. I brought Mary Ellen into the room and asked for her help in painting a picture of one of the trees outside the window. She shrugged and started in on the project. An hour later, a beautiful, detailed tree was displayed on the canvas. "Wow! I didn't think Mary Ellen could paint anymore!" one of the staff members said. "Did anyone give her a canvas to see if she actually could?" I asked.

One of the biggest obstacles to getting their loved ones with dementia to participate in activities is the reluctance of caregivers (both professional and family) to take the first step in choosing something with which to engage their person with dementia. When I was walking around the inside of a craft store one time, picking up activity items for my residents at the care community where I worked, I overheard a woman tell another one, "Yeah, the woman I look after has dementia, but I have no idea what to do with her!" I couldn't help myself and rounded the corner. I apologized for the interruption and explained what I did for a living. I then asked this woman what her client used to enjoy doing. "She used to be a hairdresser, but, of course, she can't do that anymore," the woman explained. "Why not?" I asked. I suggested she pick up a dummy and a couple of wigs. "Could you ask for her help styling wigs?" I asked. It was an off-the-cuff idea, but I felt confident that it could work. There is really no wrong way to use a job or lifestyle to develop an activity for a person with dementia—it just needs to be done in the first place.

PART III

ACTIVITIES

Lifelike Dolls and Pets

Mercy's son was unsure about my suggestion that we give his mother an artificial dog. "I don't know," he said, sighing and glancing at his mother who was watching TV in the other room. "What if she doesn't like it? Or what if she thinks it's silly that we're bringing her a toy?" he asked. "That's why we are going to give her the opportunity to tell us what she thinks about it," I explained. "We aren't going to tell her what kind of dog it is—we're just going to let her tell us. And I have the perfect dog for her."

I ran out to my car, currently parked in front of my client's house. Maybe it was a little odd, but I always kept a Memorable Pet dog in the trunk of my car. I would've kept it in the backseat, but, really, the dog looked so real I was afraid someone might try to break my window on a hot day to "rescue" the animal.

"Mercy, what do you think about this?" I asked, offering the 97-year-old woman a stuffed animal. "Oh, look at him," she grinned back. "Is that your dog?" Mercy asked. "Well, I'm hoping you can help me take care of him. Do you think you can help me with that?" I replied. Mercy nodded. "I love dogs!" she exclaimed, smiling and holding out her hands to receive the puppy.

It was official: Mercy loved it. She often asked me to carry him into the next room with us when it was time for her to eat lunch. "He's going to cry from the living room," Mercy explained. "He's going to wonder where we went."

I worked with Mercy and her son for the remainder of her life. I'll never forget what her son told me at her funeral service: "I buried her with the dog," he said, smiling sadly. "I knew she'd want it beside her forever."

There are so many amazing stories about older adults with dementia interacting with babies and animals (figure 11.1). I regularly brought therapy-certified dogs into the dementia care communities where I worked. I also loved taking my residents to visit local preschools and

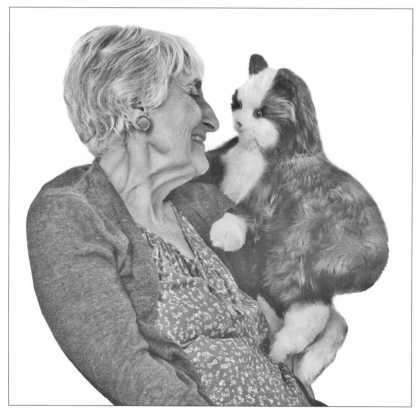

Figure 11.1. Stuffed animals and baby dolls are an easy and reliable way to provide interaction for people living with dementia. Used with permission of Memorable Pets.com.

watching them interact with the young children there. Even though these events were always beautiful and exciting, they were hard to plan. Occasionally, they were actually impossible to plan: some people with dementia cannot easily leave their homes or communities, and it can

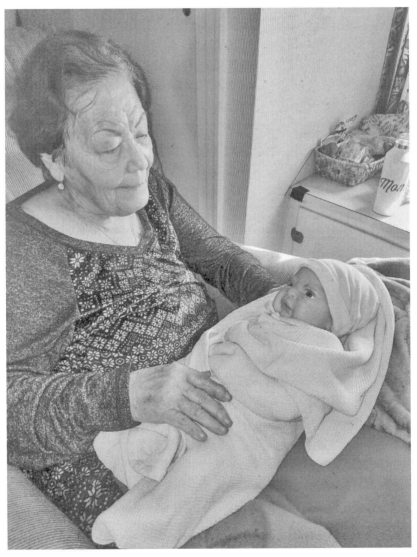

Figure 11.2. Dolls are an inexpensive way to make someone feel connected and safe. Used with permission of MemorablePets.com.

be challenging to get kids to come in for visits. The reason baby dolls and stuffed animals end up being so helpful in dementia care is that they are easy, reliable, and always present when you want them to be.

There's even scientific support for this. Since 1980, there have been 247 research papers published examining the use of what is called "doll therapy" with people with dementia. In 2017, a group of scientists conducted a review of this research (Ng, Ho, Koh, Tan, & Chan). The results of the twelve studies included in their review suggested that doll therapy made patients with dementia happier, more communicative, and even more social. According to these studies, dementia can make someone feel vulnerable and frightened, especially when they find themselves in new or threatening environments (and it is common for people with damaged short-term memory to perceive their environments as new and threatening); in these circumstances, dolls provide a source of security and connection that gives adults with dementia comfort and makes them feel less anxious. Although I do not like to ever compare older adults to children, in this instance, just as a doll can help a child who becomes anxious and worried when their parents leave, so too can it do the same for an adult with dementia. If a doll can help someone feel more connected and safe, providing one seems like an easy and inexpensive way to do so (figure 11.2).

IN A COMMUNITY SETTING

"Oh, hello, babies!" Danielle cried, reaching her arms into the crib. She picked up one of the baby dolls and held it to her chest, bouncing it lightly. "Hi, honey," she cooed softly. "How was your nap?"

I had recently purchased a full-size crib online for the skilled nursing facility's "nursery" space. I knew immediately what I was looking for, so finding the materials wasn't difficult. Really, the only difficult piece was convincing the maintenance team to set the crib up for me. "I haven't built a crib in thirty years," one of the guys said, shaking his head and laughing. "This is really weird. Do you think the residents are going to go for this?" he asked.

Indeed, they went for it. The residents loved the transformation of this sitting area turned nursery. We purchased a rocking chair, a crib, and "welcome baby!" decor. The space was transformed into something new and fresh, and the residents came in to visit the babies. A number of the residents immediately took to the babies, so much so that we had to purchase two more to meet the demand.

Danielle had previously spent most of her days walking the hallways and wringing her hands anxiously. She had a habit of folding up all of her belongings into her bedsheets and then slinging them over her shoulder like a heavy knapsack. Danielle was very tactile and also very focused on leaving the community as soon as possible. "I have to get home!" she'd say, sighing. "My kids are waiting for me to make dinner!"

The baby dolls were a perfect fit: not only did they meet Danielle's need for tactile stimulation but they also kept her mind occupied. Now instead of trying to leave, Danielle was focused on the crib. This shift in focus provided her—and the staff members—a great deal of calm.

A best practice is to create a space for the pets or dolls that is unique and draws residents in. For example, dedicating a room to be the "nursery" or "pet shop" is a great way to invite interest. Set up a crib, a rocking chair, or a pet bed to make clear the purpose of the space. Particularly if the room is being newly used for this purpose, begin by adding a music player to the space: it really helps to draw residents in when they can hear something happening in the room. Don't be afraid to invite people into the space either. "Come see this new nursery we have!" you may suggest to a resident walking by. Recognize that it may take a few days for residents to begin entering the room on their own.

I have found that spaces that are unoccupied or not given a clearly defined reason for existing may go unnoticed by many people with dementia. It may take a few days for people to start using the room again once you've redone it.

I love bringing baby dolls and stuffed animals into care community settings. Sometimes, though, it takes a bit of convincing: the communities aren't always thrilled about introducing "toys" to their residents. Let's cover some of the myths you may hear when discussing baby dolls and stuffed animals in a community setting.

"It isn't dignified"

As long as the person with dementia likes the doll or animal, it is indeed dignified. For many people with dementia, the object becomes real, and this makes the individual feel useful and important: they are caring for something or someone else again! We take things from people with cognitive impairments such as their car keys, their ability to live independently, and their cell phones only because we have to. The one thing we don't need to take is their sense of purpose and importance in the world. By giving someone a baby doll or stuffed animal, we give them the ability to do something important.

"We've already tried it"

I once had a staff member at an assisted living community tell me that they had already tried baby dolls and they didn't work. Upon investigating this original attempt, I found that the baby dolls they'd used had not looked real: they were plastic, hard, and small. No one, not even someone deep into dementia, would mistake these babies for real. Although the community had tried it, they had not executed the attempt correctly. They were also putting the dolls into residents' hands, without further instruction, or were leaving them in various rooms, hoping their residents would stumble on them. It is critically important to introduce the baby dolls effectively: make them readily available and ask the residents what they think of the babies. For this particular community, I decided to try again with more realistic-looking dolls and had a lot of success.

"We can't keep the dolls or pets clean enough"

Different companies have different policies and practices regarding the cleaning and maintenance of the baby dolls and pets. Some stuffed animals, depending on the material they are made of, can be tossed into a garment bag and then into the washing machine. Later, they can be left to air dry. Robot toys need to be wiped clean with a disinfectant wipe between users. It is important to keep the pets and babies clean, but it may also be easier to purchase interested residents their own pet or baby. Although these still need to be washed occasionally, it facilitates infection control when the dolls aren't being shared between different people.

"They are too expensive"

One of the first "pets" created for people with dementia was PARO. PARO is a seal that moves, coos, and responds to touch. It is adorable and very popular but has a high price point. While PARO is unique, there are other pets and baby dolls that do not cost nearly as much money. Memorable Pets sells many of their pets for less than $40 a pet. They also feature baby dolls on their site that range in price from low to very high. I have been known to shop Amazon for realistic-looking baby dolls and have found a number of options for under $40 a doll. The community's monetary investment in baby dolls and pets can be really high or fairly low, but no matter the actual cost, the items, as long as they are realistic looking, are always worth it.

"One of our residents will hog all the babies or pets"

This is something I have heard a number of times, and sometimes it's true. If that is the case, however, it is easily solvable: provide enough pets and baby dolls for the person who really enjoys them. Dress all the dolls in a particular color or put little bows in the dogs' hair. If one of the residents is hoarding the items, they will probably keep them in their own room. It will typically be easy to slip in and remove some of the dolls or pets that don't belong to them. Of course, arguing is not an option. We never want to say, "That's not yours!" Instead, wait until the resident is at a meal, go into their room, and take out the pets or dolls that belong to other residents. It is very unlikely that, at this stage in their dementia, they will discover that one of their dolls is missing.

Conclusion

No matter what the argument against using baby dolls or pets is, I always believe that it's worth a try. Even if a large majority of the residents don't enjoy them, if one person does, it is a success. Could utilizing baby dolls or pets invite more drama, such as residents fighting over them? Absolutely. However, the benefits almost always outweigh the negative outcomes.

AT HOME

Vince's wife was excited: she'd finally found something that might keep him occupied during the day. "He gets bored," she said, approaching me after my caregiver class. "I'm going to purchase one of those Memorable Pets you mentioned today," she said, smiling. "I really think he's going to like it."

The next week, Vince's wife returned to class, victorious. "He loves that cat," she said, running up to me and taking my hands in hers. "Thank you so much for talking about those pets. I don't think he believes the cat is real, but . . . it doesn't seem to matter! He loves it, anyway."

A best practice, when using baby dolls or pets at home, is to set up a space in the house where they can "live." This space doesn't have to be a whole room or even half a room: you can easily set up a pet bed on an end table in your living room. The main point of having a dedicated space is to prevent the pets or baby dolls from getting lost. They have a "home" to return to, which comes in particularly handy if the person living with dementia needs a break from the doll.

Having worked in home care environments and directly with families of those with dementia, I have heard a number of arguments against using pets or dolls in the home. Most of these arguments are based on myths that someone has heard. Let's review some of the myths about using dolls at home.

"What if she doesn't like it?"

To this question, my response is usually, "Well, let's give it a try." One of the more challenging aspects of dementia is that people with it tend to have poor short-term memories. But one of the benefits of dementia is that because people with it have poor short-term memories, we can try things more than once. It is nearly impossible to conclude that someone will like or dislike a doll without trying it first. The good news is that you can always try again later if it doesn't work the first time.

"They are too expensive"

As long as the doll or pet is realistic, it doesn't really matter where you find it. Memorable Pets has a nice selection of pets and dolls for very reasonable prices. Ageless Innovation makes robotic cats and dogs that they sell at a higher price point but still within a very reasonable range. I recommend doing some shopping around to find the best deal, but you do not have to break the bank to purchase a realistic-looking pet or doll.

"The client already has ten baby dolls and doesn't think that they are real"

The issue may be that the baby dolls do not look or feel real enough. Cabbage Patch dolls or a similar item, for example, are great for kids, but they do not look realistic enough for adults. The goal in finding a doll or pet is to find something that looks real and promotes dignity and respect for the person with dementia.

Of course, it could also be that the individual just doesn't believe that dolls are real, and that's okay, too! Again, whatever they think about it is the right answer. But even if the person has not reacted positively before, it's almost always worth another try.

"He might think it's real and then won't interact with his real great-grandchildren"

This was a particularly odd interaction I had with a client's daughter. She was very fixated on the fact that her father might become so attached to the doll that he would neglect his own great-grandchildren when they came over. We introduced the doll anyway, and he loved it. Although he did also interact with and enjoy his great-grandchildren when they came over, our client's daughter was not convinced and remained ambivalent. She ended up returning the baby doll to us.

The great thing about the baby doll was that it was real to him, as were his actual great-grandchildren. They shared the same weight in his mind, and that was okay. He treated both the baby doll and his real great-grandchildren with love and affection and wanted to hold both of them constantly. It did not really matter who was real and who was fake: he wasn't going to drop either of them from his arms, and he believed them both to be very important.

"She might get too focused on it and then won't eat or do other activities"

It's possible that the individual living with dementia will become very attached to, and fixated on, a pet or baby doll. This is actually good news, and it is also easily addressed if the person becomes too focused on the item. A great way to take the doll from the individual with dementia is to suggest that it "needs a nap" or "needs to go to the bathroom."

Conclusion

There is never really a good reason to avoid trying something that the person living with dementia may enjoy. The worst thing that can happen is that they don't like it or are confused as to why you are showing it to them. Asking "What do you think about this?" makes the original introduction a lot easier. By using this phrasing, you are not inserting your own view on what the pet or doll may mean to the individual. Let the person with dementia tell you what they think of the doll and then go along with that reality.

Exercise

THE IMPORTANCE OF EXERCISE

It was my first time meeting Chris, and his daughter had requested that our home care agency do some exercise with him. Specifically, she wanted us to walk with him around the block, and maybe even take his small dog with us. I didn't know much about Chris before I went to visit him, although his daughter had mentioned that he "had some trouble with his memory." Upon visiting, though, I realized that his daughter had underestimated her father's condition. Chris had mild-to-moderate dementia and trouble walking even a few feet inside the house. His daughter had clearly overestimated Chris's ability to walk around the neighborhood safely. I wanted to fulfill her wishes, but I also wanted to ensure that we were doing the safest thing for Chris.

"Let's do some warm-up exercises before we go on our walk," I suggested. "Oh, I like stretching! I ran track in high school," he said, smiling back. I had a couple of goals with regard to the stretching. For one, I wanted to see how Chris would do with following instructions. I also wanted to see if he would struggle to complete these exercises, which would tell me a lot about his ability to walk outside. After years of leading group exercise in dementia care communities, one-on-one exercise instruction came easy to me: I'd found that even the most advanced of my residents were able to mimic my movements and follow along while we did our morning stretching.

As I had done when leading group sessions in the past, I stayed seated while doing each stretch. Chris was able to sit across from me and mimic my movements with ease. Our time exercising also gave us a chance to talk more: Chris was able to stretch and chat with me about the photos hanging on his wall. After I felt a little more confident about his ability to walk safely, we went outside. Chris and I only walked up and back about two blocks, but he was clearly happy with this success. "I love getting exercise during the day," he told me as we headed back inside.

One of my favorite things to do with people living with dementia is exercise. Exercise can be anything from morning stretches to a game of balloon toss. For the most part, exercise involves almost zero setup and almost no extra materials. In this chapter, I review some exercises, stretching, and physical games that you can do in home or community settings. The only difference between in-home and community settings is the group size. From one-on-one to groups of fifteen or more, the only real adjustment you need to make is how loud you speak. I have found that, even for individuals who are advanced in their dementia, exercise comes easily: most everyone is able to mimic and follow along.

It is also important that a physician sign off on the participation of individuals in these exercise regimens. If you notice someone struggling or looking like they are in pain, instruct them to stop the exercise. Make sure that in a group setting you are watching for extra confusion or pain. Quietly escort someone who looks uncomfortable to another room without disrupting the group.

SETTING THE SCENE

Time of Day

Time of day is perhaps the most important factor when it comes to exercise programs for people who have dementia. For example, when I ran stretching and warm-up programs in dementia care communities, I would always schedule them for first thing in the morning and then again after lunch. I found that postmeal exercise was a great way to wake my residents back up after they had eaten. It doesn't have to last a long time either: even just twenty minutes of stretching is perfect. It can be a segue to a new activity or it can be an activity in and of itself. When you engage people with dementia in more physical activities, such as a game of balloon toss, limit it to less than forty-five minutes. Most people will become tired or bored if the game goes much longer than that. The goal is to get people engaged, ensure they have fun, and then stop when the energy starts to wane.

To Sit or to Stand

Do you want to sit or stand while running your exercise program? It is really a matter of preference, but I prefer to sit. I think it's easier to show the exercise that your group will be doing when you are in the same position that they are. Since your individual or individuals with dementia will be sitting, I think it makes the most sense to sit along with them. It's easiest for them to mimic when they don't have to think about the exercise from a standing position.

Group Size

Group size will vary depending on your setting. If you are working with one person, sit them across from you, facing you directly. If you are working with a larger group, gather them around you in a half circle.

It's important that you are able to see each person and that they are each able to see you. In a group, you may need to offer some individual attention without calling anyone out too explicitly. I found that walking up to people and touching them softly worked well. For more extroverted individuals, I would call their name with a smile: "Keep going, Joyce! You're doing great!"

Background Noise

Music in the background can be nice, but it can also be distracting. You may end up singing instead of stretching, so pick music without lyrics if you want to play something in the background. I like to pick a spot to exercise that is away from distractions. If you are running the group in a senior living community, you probably face a lot of potential distractions: staff members walking by, medications being passed out, and family members stopping in to visit. When one person with dementia becomes distracted by something, it tends to be contagious. Distractions are also another reason that you want to keep your exercise program relatively short.

Getting Them Engaged

Hearing the word "exercise" makes a lot of people cringe. I have found that asking individuals living with dementia if they want to exercise does not often receive the desired response. Instead, I often skip the question. "Come with me" or "Let's sit here" is usually how I start my exercise program. I then start an exercise and tell the person or people to follow along. Some individuals need more encouragement to start or keep going, so add in a lot of praise. "Great job!" or "Just like that!" are fantastic phrases to use. People are much more likely to keep going if they feel encouraged and positive about what they are doing.

Working with a Disruptive Party

One of my favorite residents at my first community was also one of the more extroverted individuals that lived there. Sheri didn't speak, but she generally understood what was happening around her and always wanted to be involved. She had a tendency to walk into a game that involved a ball, grab the ball, and then walk away with it. Sheri did this with full knowledge that she had interrupted the game—she enjoyed the attention that she gained when everyone yelled at her to return the ball. Eventually, knowing that this was Sheri's goal and that there was really no way to prevent her from accomplishing it once she was in the room, I had other staff members keep her occupied in a different space of the building.

EXAMPLES OF EXERCISES AND PHYSICAL GAMES

Mimicked Stretching

I have found that people living with dementia mimic others very well (figure 12.1). Even for individuals who are advanced in their dementia, watching and following others is far from a lost skill. Sit across from your individual or group, and announce that it's time to wake up a little bit. Announce each stretch while you are demonstrating it, and then do it along with everyone else. Here are some easy, seated stretches to try:

- While sitting, stretch your legs out straight and touch your toes.

- Rotate your ankles.

- Flex your foot and point your toes.

- Stretch your arms up in the air.

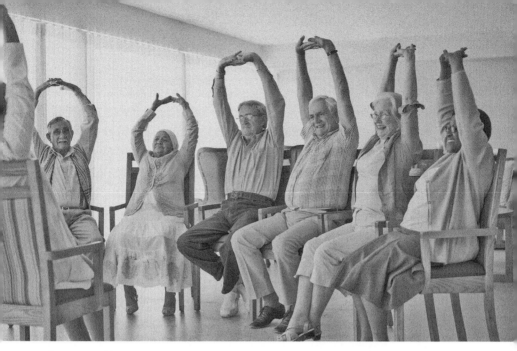

Figure 12.1. Mimicked stretching can even engage individuals with advanced dementia

- Hold your arms out to the side and rotate them in small circles, clockwise and counterclockwise.

- Slowly roll your head around on your neck.

- Smile and then frown, smile and then frown.

Weight Training

Who says that people with cognitive impairments can't do weight training? These weights should not be more than five pounds (figure 12.2), as this is more about exercise and stretching than it is about gaining muscle. This is a great program to introduce if the person or people with dementia feel like they aren't being challenged enough with normal stretching. This can also be an excellent program for individuals who used to lift weights but stopped once their cognitive issues progressed.

Figure 12.2. Adding hand weights to a stretching routine can help people with dementia who don't feel challenged enough

Balloon Toss

If you've ever been to a senior living community, you have probably seen residents play this game (figure 12.3). It can be used one-on-one or in a group setting and requires minimal setup. You will want an inflated balloon (or two) and maybe some foam pool noodles, although those are optional. (If you have a particularly rowdy group, skip the pool noodles: I've watched one too many fights break out over someone getting accidentally tapped, unexpectedly, with a noodle.) Explain that the goal of the game is to keep the balloon in the air as long as possible. Hands, pool noodles, feet, and even tops of heads are useful during this game. Turn on some background music and begin by tossing the balloon to someone.

If this is one-on-one, sit across from the individual. If this is a group, gather everyone in a circle. In large groups, to increase the amount of time that the balloon stays afloat, you may want to ensure that the more physically active residents are seated next to residents who aren't as

Figure 12.3. Balloon toss is an easy activity that can engage small and large groups

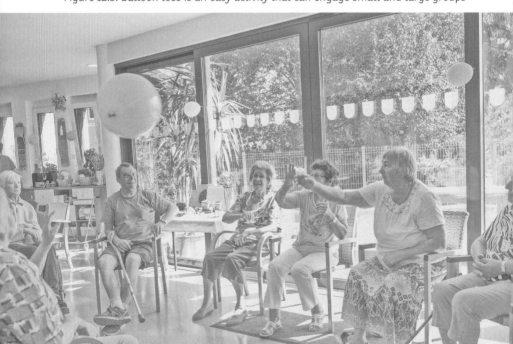

physically active. This also prevents you from running around the room for the entire game.

Seated Soccer/Football

While I call this "soccer," or "football," it isn't exactly akin to either American soccer or football. There aren't goal posts set up, so the only goal is to pass the ball using your feet for as long as possible. I recommend a soft, large ball—something similar to a beach ball works best. Encourage everyone to try and keep the ball on the ground. This provides great leg exercise and involves minimal risks, since participants are sitting during the game.

If you are hosting this game inside of someone's house, ensure that fragile lamps and items are out of the way, even if you feel confident that there's no way the ball will go airborne. And again, if this is a group, ensure that residents with differing abilities are seated next to each other. You don't want an entire group of strong kickers across from a group of individuals who can barely move the ball. I also recommend filling the gaps between chairs with cones so that you are not chasing the ball everywhere.

Basketball

While you are welcome to try setting up a basketball hoop on the back of a door, I find that most seated individuals cannot toss a ball that high (figure 12.4). Unlike traditional basketball, this game features a basket on the floor. Most any ball and basket will do; if you're in someone's house, a laundry basket is perfect. I recommend finding a ball that fits in two hands, as it is less likely to go missing or flying across the room in the wrong direction. Participants can toss it or bounce it into the basket.

This game has been incredibly popular everywhere that I've used it. In groups, my residents cheer and egg each other on. They even clap

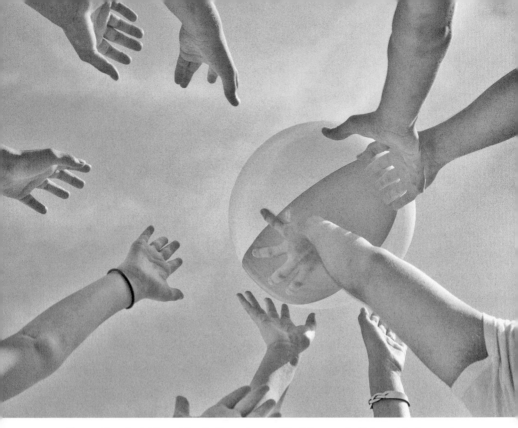

Figure 12.4. Activities with a ball can be modified for people living with dementia

when someone makes a basket. I like this game because you can easily adjust the level of difficulty. For example, if you have an individual who has great hand-eye coordination, move the basket farther away. If you have someone who can barely toss the ball, surreptitiously move the basket closer to them. It's easy to make everyone feel proud and successful during this game.

Bowling

Most any toy store, online or otherwise, will have a small bowling set. Get your group gathered around the pins in a circle or set your individual up across from them. If it's a group, let people have three tries to knock down all the pins. I will admit that this is not my favorite game. It involves a lot of leaning down and picking up pins for the person coordinating the game. For this reason, it is probably best played one-on-one.

Bag Toss

Bag toss is another wildly popular game that I've tried both with my residents and in a home care setting. It's easy and involves very little setup. If you happen to have small cornhole boards, you can use these. You could also use any basket or other wooden board with a hole or holes cut into it. At one community, we lacked a wooden board, so I found three different size baskets. These worked just as well and our residents enjoyed competing to get the bag into the smallest basket.

Table Ball / Table Pong

This game is perfect for before or after meals, but be aware that it can get pretty boisterous. Gather around a table and try to keep the ball on the table. Alternatively, set up cups on the table and fill them with water. Use a ping pong ball and take turns trying to land a ball in the cup. While most people normally play this game with beer, that usually isn't a great option in this type of setting. Make sure that everyone knows the water in the cups isn't for drinking: it gets dirty pretty quickly!

SUMMARY

There are many studies indicating the importance of exercise for persons with dementia. Changes such as fewer falls, better sleep, more positive mood and better overall mental health, and reduced risk for sundowning have all been outcomes associated with appropriate physical exercise (Whitlatch & Orsulic-Jeras, 2018). The great thing about all of the ideas I have described is that they can be modified based on group size and ease. When I would begin my design for an activity calendar, I'd pick up to two different physical activities for each day. I really felt like it got my residents' moods and spirits up after they'd done some exercise. Even some light stretching after a meal can work wonders for a person with dementia.

Music

I think that nearly everyone has seen the YouTube videoclip about a man living with dementia named Henry. He becomes almost miraculously lucid after someone puts headphones on him and plays the music he loves. In fact, Henry goes from being nearly nonverbal to talking about "sharing the love" and how much music means to him. The changes in his whole appearance—he begins to smile and gets animated and excited—as well as his sudden ability to speak brings tears to the eyes of anyone watching his transformation. This video was made popular by a program called "Music and Memory" that provides adults living with dementia music players with their favorite songs.

Music has long been used as a tool for working with persons with dementia. Music has been found to reduce anxiety, to encourage interaction, to reduce agitation (Sung, Lee, Li, & Watson, 2012), and to increase cooperation in persons with dementia (Clark, Lipe, & Bilbrey, 1998). Throughout the chapters on activities, I've even suggested that background music can help calm and set the mood for everything from meal times to participation in multisensory rooms. Even without the research to back up the argument that music has a positive effect, it's clear the impact that music has. I myself have a workout playlist that I've been adding to since I was a teenager. I chose every song on that playlist for the energy that it gives me when it comes on. We are all familiar with the way music makes us feel. When we're depressed, we want music that matches our mood. When we are cleaning up the house for a party later that evening, we probably want upbeat, energetic tunes. People living with dementia are just as affected by music as people without any cognitive impairments.

The most boring communities and houses that I've been to had their silence broken only by a television set. Even when we are shopping, we expect music: think about it—going into a completely silent store is a bizarre experience. You think, "Why is it so quiet in here?" when you can only hear the store employees chatting among themselves. People living with dementia likewise feel uneasy in the midst of silence. The progressively lowered stress threshold model proposed by G. R. Hall and Kathleen Buckwalter (1987) explains that dementia impacts the ability to handle stressors that make people with dementia anxious and agitated. Music can help drown out or override some external stressors while allowing more pleasant memories to be recalled.

Maybe, too, it's as simple as that listening to one's preferred music simply helps one connect to the past, thereby reducing stress and the anxiety that develops as a result of dementia (Gerdner, 2000). The key here is preferred or personalized music selections. And then there are the stories of the "awakenings" that happen when persons with dementia are able to listen to music that is meaningful to them (as in the case of Henry).

The good news is that introducing music isn't hard to do. Adding a CD player to a room, piping in music over the speakers via Bluetooth connected to a smartphone, or putting earphones on someone's ears is easy. The most challenging part, really, is finding music that everyone likes. This is, of course, much more difficult when there is more than one person listening. When working in senior living communities, I opt for music of a certain era that I assume everyone will at least accept, if not deeply enjoy.

MUSICAL INSTRUMENTS

Why music works is still largely unknown. Researchers have focused on the changes in behaviors that seem to accompany the playing of music and have not succeeded in finding out why it is so effective. People living with dementia who had played musical instruments earlier in their lives are often able to still remember how to play the instruments because the long-term memory, especially procedural memory, appears to be less affected by dementia (as compared to short-term memories). So when musical instruments are reintroduced to them, they become engaged and interested. There's also some theoretical support for the more positive effect of live music over recorded music. Since using musical instruments increases the opportunity for interaction, it might be more beneficial than simply listening to a recording (Sherratt, Thornton, & Hatton, 2004).

The reason for the sudden "awakenings" and changes in verbal behavior that have been shown to occur is even harder to pinpoint. In recent research at the University of Utah (King et al. 2018), researchers used functional magnetic resonance imaging that showed that when a person listens to music that is personally important and memorable, a unique region of the brain and one of the last areas to be damaged by dementia (called the salience network) becomes active; the networks in that region that are responsible for paying attention to certain things in particular are activated. Even more interesting is that researchers have found that listening to personally meaningful music (compared to silence or listening to music played in reverse and rendered meaningless) causes multiple regions of the brain in this network to work together. So that even though dementia damages certain regions of the brain, those less affected areas are recruited and work together to increase a person's coherence, clarity, or "wakefulness." We have to be careful to not get too excited about these findings, because only a very few people were studied, but this research has given us some insight as to how the brain might be related to the "awakenings" that occur in some persons with dementia after listening to music that is meaning-ful to them.

One of the most well-known music programs out today, the Music and Memory program, gives iPods to long-term care facilities and other elder care workers, including family caregivers, to use with their patients or loved ones with dementia. They currently are being used in more than three thousand elder care facilities in the United States and abroad (musicandmemory.org/about/mission-and-vision). They also provide training in how to use the iPods and other devices and how to create personalized music lists in order to help people with dementia "reconnect with the world through music-triggered memories" (Cohen, Post, Lo, Lombardo, & Pfeffer, 2018). Through the organization's website, you can even donate used iPods that will be given away to those who need them. Recently, a study found that the Music and Memory program helped people with advanced dementia swallow (Cohen et al. 2018). Keep in mind that in the advanced stages, persons with dementia may have a hard time with swallowing, eating, and drinking, resulting in significant weight loss and risk for dehydration. Care providers might have to use other, sometimes unpleasant, ways to introduce liquids and food, and so if music can help with swallowing, its benefits are that much greater.

TYPES OF MUSIC

The type of music you're going to use really depends on what your goals are. If your goal is to help a group engage in an activity together (like eating a meal), then quiet background music, preferably without lyrics, can help create a calming environment that will not take away from the task at hand. However, the best music for a person with dementia is typically music that is personally meaningful to them, and so in group settings, this means that the music has to be delivered personally via headphones hooked up to some source of music. Keep in mind that those tiny ear buds that are so popular these days probably will be too hard to use, so it's likely that you'll want to use headphones you can adjust the volume on. You don't want the music to be too loud and uncomfortable to listen to.

There are also issues around the use of equipment in larger care communities. Just as with dolls and stuffed animals, iPods, headphones, and other equipment might be taken by the residents with dementia. The best thing to do is go into residents' rooms and return the equipment, but that means that an already overburdened staff is now responsible for expensive equipment.

If your primary purpose in using music is to increase engagement or even autobiographical recall, personalized music is the way to go. A 2013 study found that when people living with dementia could self-select the music they were going to listen to, they used more words when they spoke and that rather than speak a series of unrelated words that is typical in persons with more advanced dementia, they spoke words that were more connected and had more meaning (Haj, Clement, Fasotti, & Allain, 2013). All of the research about music and "awakenings" has supported this. And it makes sense. If I love the music of the 1960s, why would swing music have any meaning for me?

14

Technology

I have split this chapter into two parts: "When Technology Is a Good Idea" and "When Technology Is a Bad Idea." I've done this because we can't talk about technology and dementia care without discussing the inherent problems in mixing the two. I have a saying that goes like this: "No amount of technology can replace human caregiving." This is an important concept for everyone who cares for a loved one with dementia at home or works in a dementia care community to understand. I have often seen families of people with dementia rely on technology to provide care for their loved ones. GPS tracking watches, cameras, medication reminders, tablets, fall-alert technology, and other devices become crutches for desperate caregivers. "Mom is safe at home alone because she has an alert necklace," I've occasionally heard family members state. The problem is this: an alert necklace doesn't work if you take it off or don't know how to press the button for assistance.

All of that said, technology can also provide wonderful, happy things in dementia caregiving. Technology ought not to be used in the hope that it will allow a person with dementia to remain safe if left alone for extended periods of time, but it can enhance the lives of adults with dementia. For example, one of the most popular examples of a piece of technology that has proved very effective in dementia care is a robotic seal named PARO that responds to touch and sound. In this chapter, we will review a number of dementia-disrupting programs and apps. When used appropriately, technology can improve the lives of caregivers and people living with dementia.

WHEN TECHNOLOGY IS A BAD IDEA

Because I work in dementia care and make that known online, I often hear from people in the tech industry. Once a month or so, I will receive a message that goes like this: "Hi, I've built an app that helps people with dementia. Can I send you more information so that you can review it for me?" When I first started in this business, I'd review every app that came my way. What I began to find, however, was that I just ended up disappointing the tech people who sent me their apps.

One was an application that worked with your tablet. It was a "memory clock" that not only told you what time it was but also reminded you of any events that were coming up. There was nothing particularly wrong with the application itself, but it certainly wasn't dementia-friendly: you had to know how the tablet worked to find out what day and time it was! If you forget to charge the tablet or forgot to look at it, the app was useless. And that is the whole trouble with dementia: people with dementia are not sure what they don't know. I told the man who sent me the tablet that I was sorry but that it just didn't make sense for people with dementia. "This would be fine if it was used for someone in a very, very early stage of dementia," I wrote to him. "Or if it was used as a supplemental piece on top of actual caregiving. My concern is that a lot of families are going to see this and think that it can be an adequate substitute for supervision."

Some families hear about alert necklaces and GPS locators and think that it's the answer to all of their concerns: now their loved one with dementia can be safe at home alone. However, this just isn't true. I remember going to a client's house one time to see how he was doing. My client's daughter thought that she'd had it all figured out: she'd outfitted the whole house with cameras and put a GPS locator watch on her father's wrist. She'd labeled all of the cabinets and put notes on the doors that read "Dad, don't go outside." She meant well, but she was trying to solve a challenging problem with the wrong kind of elbow grease. Her dad didn't need more technology or notes; he just needed more actual caregiving. While the notes and the tech made her feel better, her father never read the notes and often took off the GPS watch. When she was at work, she couldn't always check the cameras either, so it was easy for her father to wander outside without anyone stopping him.

There's a terrible, false sense of security that technology seems to give caregivers. I think it's because a lot of programs or apps are advertised as a "solution" rather than an "addition" to care. I'm not suggesting you avoid using technological advances to help care for people with dementia, but I am suggesting that they cannot be the *only* thing that you utilize. While alert necklaces and various cameras and GPS systems are excellent ways to enhance the care we provide for people with dementia, they aren't enough on their own. In the end, they can't replace human-to-human contact. Unless something significant changes in the coming years and robots with artificial intelligence become popular (and affordable!), we have nothing that compares to human caregiving. There is no substitute for good, reliable, hands-on care in dementia.

WHEN TECHNOLOGY IS A GOOD IDEA

When we think about technology and dementia, we need to consider more examples than an alert necklace or a well-placed stair chair lift. What about the products that enhance the lives of people with dementia by engaging them? Tablet or smartphone apps are a great way to engage people with dementia, as long as the applications are easy to use and understand. There are also a number of interactive programs that have been expressly built for people with dementia. Some communities in the Netherlands have pioneered highly interactive programs for their residents with dementia.

Tablet Applications

Look for apps that don't require a lot of instructions or buttons (figure 14.1). There are a number of applications available for people wanting to "brain train" (Luminosity, Elevate), but these are better for people who don't have dementia or who are in very early stages of cognitive loss. The goal of a good app for someone with dementia is not to "fix" their dementia or try to improve their cognition; instead, the goal should be to engage them and enhance their life in a fun way. Here are some tablet- or smartphone-based apps that I recommend.

Virtual Aquarium

An aquarium, calming and colorful, without all of the mess! There are numerous applications that offer a chance to care for an aquarium on your tablet or smartphone, so they do not need to be reviewed here. No matter which program you choose, your loved one with dementia

Figure 14.1. Using a tablet is a great way to engage people with dementia if the apps are easy to use and understand

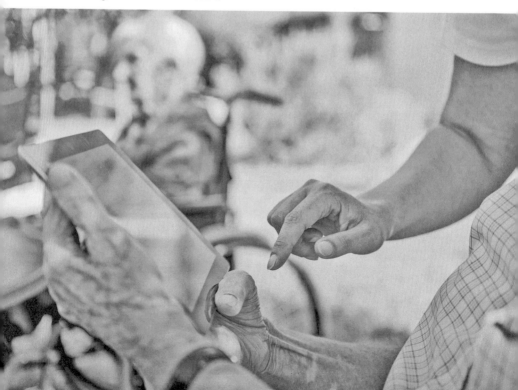

can have an opportunity to care for fish without all of the challenges that come with having an actual tank. This type of app is great for stress relief, especially for people who love fish (figure 14.2).

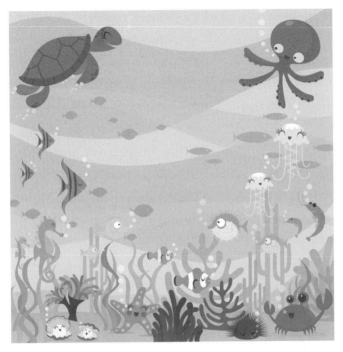

Figure 14.2. Virtual aquariums relieve stress without the mess that comes with owning real fish

Virtual Pets

When I was a kid, there were these great little toys called Tamagotchis. They were virtual key ring–sized games—far too small for my eyes, now, I'm sure—that allowed you to take care of a cat, dog, dinosaur, you name it. You'd feed the pet, take it for walks, and make sure it slept well. There were even options for you to sync your Tamagotchi with your friend's Tamagotchi, thereby giving you an opportunity to turn it into a multi-player event. We absolutely adored these things, and I feel confident in saying that we also annoyed our parents by asking them to "babysit" our Tamagotchis while we went in the pool or out for a bike ride.

This technology is now completely outdated, although a new generation of Tamagotchis has been introduced, and there are better, more vision-friendly options for your loved one with dementia. As with virtual aquariums, there are too many options to name, but apps like Daily Kitten, where you care for a virtual cat, or Pet City, where you can choose from a number of pets are popular (figure 14.3).

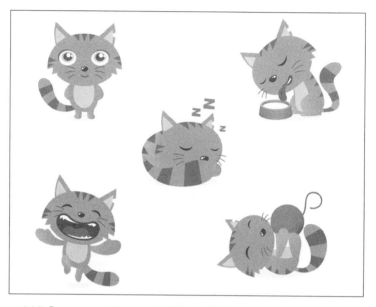

Figure 14.3. Some apps allow people living with dementia to care for virtual pets

Coloring, Painting, or Word Search Apps

Painting and coloring apps provide an opportunity for people living with dementia to create art without caregivers having to worry about the cleanup. It's Never 2 Late is an interactive program with a number of different applications. Painting apps are available on any smartphone or tablet. If your loved one likes to paint or draw, these apps can provide a lot of calm, especially on trips or in waiting rooms. It is much easier to carry a tablet than to carry a coloring book and markers everywhere you go. The same goes for word search apps or crossword puzzles. If you have someone who enjoys brain games, this may be a perfect fit.

Balloon Popping Apps

It seems almost silly, but a great, task-oriented app is one where users can pop balloons, bubble wrap, or complete another repetitive motion. Balloon Popper by Spigo allows you to do just that. It's easy to follow along and easy to set up. Just as with the other recommendations in this chapter, there are a number of options out there to choose from, so explore them in order to find the right app for your loved one or client.

Music and Breathing Apps

Personally, I like a nice breathing app. It sounds almost too simple to even be an app, but it's not: it is an app that encourages deep, calm breathing. We all know that there's a positive correlation between emotional calm and guided breathing or meditation. These applications provide a visualizer that demonstrates the rate at which you should inhale and exhale. Apps like these are perfect for combatting sundowning, particularly if you and the person with dementia you are caring for can practice breathing together.

Interactive Programs

It's Never 2 Late

My first nine-to-five job in dementia care was at a Brookdale community in North Carolina. Not long after I started, we received a system called It's Never 2 Late. Brookdale had purchased the program and a few extra components that could be used with it. It's Never 2 Late is a program that runs through the community's television and also connects via USB cable to a number of physical devices, such as a music-making machine and actual bike pedals (figure 14.4). With the help of the person running the program, participants are able to do a number of different activities that are already programmed into the system. We played music trivia, made Skype calls to residents' families, and created pages for each resident with their various likes and favorite programs.

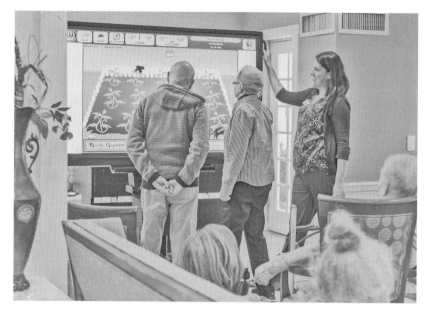

Figure 14.4. Participants using It's Never 2 Late. Used with permission of It's Never 2 Late.

PARO

You can't work in dementia care without hearing about PARO, the seal that was invented by a Japanese company and that has been sold all over the world (figure 14.5). It's not cheap (it runs about $6,000 USD), but it really is adorable. It comes in a few different coat colors and interacts with its user by making cute sounds and facial expressions. It responds to touch and sound; petting PARO, for example, elicits a happy noise from the robotic animal. The company has suggested that people with dementia are happier, calmer, and more lively and interactive with others after using the robot.

Joy for All Pets

The Joy for All website advertises itself with the slogan "No vet bills, just love." Much like PARO, the pets the company sells respond to touch. Early in my career working for myself, Joy for All sent me a cat to review. I have been bringing it with me to conferences and trainings ever since, because it always gets a great response from the crowd. Many people without dementia have exclaimed, "Wow! I thought that was a real cat!" after they heard it meow from across the room (figure 14.6).

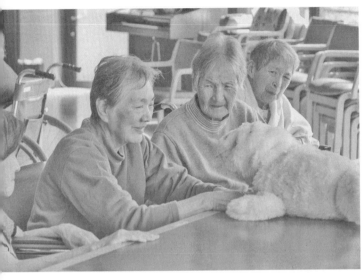

Figure 14.5 (*above*). Participant interacting with a PARO. Used with permission of the National Institute of Advanced Industrial Science and Technology (AIST), Japan.

Figure 14.6 (*right*). Stuffed animals can provide realistic engagement for people living with engagement. Used with permission of Joy for All.

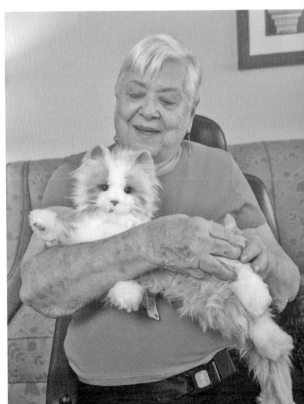

Simulations

The residents pictured in figure 14.5 are sitting in a room made to look and feel like the beach. The floor has real sand, there are heat-regulating lamps, and beach sounds are piped in over the speaker system. Another community has a ceiling simulator that displays calming nature scenes on a resident's room ceiling, which is particularly useful for bedbound individuals. While these simulations are amazing in scope, they do not have to be this elaborate. There are a number of flight and bike simulators that work on regular televisions or computer systems. The goal of the simulation is always to inspire positive feelings in the user.

COMMUNICATION

When Angela's mother had major surgery, she had to find a place for her father, who was in the early stages of Alzheimer disease, to stay for a couple of months while her mother recovered. She eventually found a room for her father in a well-thought-of facility. In order to ease the separation between her parents for these months, Angela used her computer to set up live video chats between her mother and father. But she noticed that her father just got increasingly upset seeing his wife each day and not understanding why he wasn't with her, and her mother became increasingly worried about the well-being of her husband. Angela realized that these video chats weren't doing either of her parents any good and quickly stopped arranging them.

Another interesting use of technology is for communication and connection. Using technology like Skype, FaceTime, and even Zoom to make it possible to see loved ones who aren't nearby or who are in other ways unable to be present makes sense. But as the case of Angela's parents suggests, it is important to carefully evaluate the effectiveness of such use.

APPLICATIONS FOR YOU TO USE

There are also a lot of apps that are built for caregivers to use alongside people who have dementia. These applications usually work on tablets and offer the user the ability to track and record information about clients or residents. Users are able to record information like residents' likes, dislikes, history, and more. They can also save residents' favorite music artists or clips from their favorite movies. A good example is RemindMeCare, an application developed in the UK.

CONCLUSION

In summary, there is no shortage of great technological advances that can help us enhance the lives of people with dementia. There are also a number of options to make caregiving easier, especially in home care settings. Knowing all of this, it's imperative that we use technology with the goal of enhancing caregiving rather than with the aim of attempting to erase it. Most of the new technology apps that aren't for monitoring or collecting information about someone with dementia are best used collaboratively. They're simply types of tools to help engage someone. There is still no substitute for human interaction in dementia care.

15

Holidays

The latest upcoming holiday is always a great conversation starter, even with strangers on the street. When I work hands-on with people living with dementia, I always make it a point to bring up the next holiday in conversation. It never ceases to amaze me how fantastic many people are at recounting stories etched into their long-term memories. Traditions that happen every year always make the longest-lasting impressions, so holidays are a great way to get someone talking about their past.

Holidays can also be a stressful time for families who have loved ones with dementia. Even if the person lives in a care community, should the family visit them? Should they bring the party to the person, or the person to the party? Here are a few guidelines for getting started when preparing for an upcoming holiday:

1. Try not to panic or get stressed. The more everyone around the person living with dementia is panicking, the more they will panic as well. Anxiety is contagious, especially for people living with dementia.

2. Decide if it makes more sense to bring the party to the person or the person to the party. If Grandmom gets agitated whenever she has to return to her skilled nursing facility, it's probably better not to take her out of the community in the first place. It may make more sense, in this case, to bring friends and family to her. Ask the facility if they have a common space you can borrow for the evening, and then bring a small dose of the festivities right to Grandmom.

It is generally easier to bring the party to the person with dementia, but don't forsake traditions before you need to. If everyone has been gathering at Aunt Penni's house for Christmas for the last few years, it may make sense to see if Grandmom could spend the evening there as well. If it seems like she doesn't mind the crowd or the time spent away from her house, then it is probably the best approach.

3. Limit the person's exposure time: don't let the individual living with dementia get overwhelmed by the amount of people or conversation happening at the gathering. Choose a quiet space for them to spend some time every couple hours so that they can get a break if they need it.

4. Don't plan too much. Creating a minute-by-minute outline of how the evening will look is going to cause more stress than it's worth. Instead, focus on the overall goal of the night: to create an enjoyable, welcoming space for your loved one with dementia.

5. Give the individual a task to complete. No one likes to watch everyone run around, busy with important things to do, while they sit idly. Often, we take tasks from people with dementia because we assume they won't be able to do them or that they'll take too long. Provide an easy, one-or-two-step task like folding tablecloths or arranging flowers to make them feel helpful and necessary.

6. Don't take away traditions, even if you are afraid that the person won't be able to do the task well enough. For example, if your loved one with dementia had a tradition of prepping the turkey, let them continue to prep the turkey. You can easily modify it to fit what they are currently able to do. For example, perhaps you make the stuffing ahead of time and then let them stuff the turkey.

7. Suggest that each family member wear a name tag—even if you believe that your loved one living with dementia knows everyone's name. Name tags can be disguised as a game of sorts by attaching alliterative adjectives to each person's name, such as "silly" to Sandra or "curious" to Callie. It's a great way to make the person living with dementia feel less intimidated or embarrassed if they forget a name.

8. Respect dietary changes in a way that makes the person with dementia feel included. If your aunt with dementia is on a pureed diet, offering the rest of the family the pureed sweet potatoes is also a great way to make her feel like she's not alone. Then she won't be the only person eating the puree.

You can probably think of a number of other thoughtful solutions to potential dementia-related issues when planning a holiday soirée. The key is to respect the person living with dementia and their limitations. All of the suggestions I have made can help caregivers assist the individual in an inconspicuous way.

HOLIDAY CRAFTS AND IDEAS

Log on to a site like Pinterest and you'll be inundated with holiday-themed crafts, cocktails, songs, and decor. There are probably a million different ways to engage someone living with dementia in holiday-related ways, but here we cover a few options that have worked for us. These are broken down by holiday, with a craft, entertainment, and food option for each one. Of course, there are countless holidays that we don't address here, all celebrated by different places and cultures in the world. Hopefully, these will give you a few ideas.

New Year's Eve/Day

Craft: Firework Art

Create "fireworks" on paper using only paper, paint, and a fork (figure 15.1). It's easy, fun, and always comes out looking good, so no one has to worry about "messing it up," which is a concern I've sometimes heard from clients with dementia. Ask for help with creating some decor for the upcoming holiday and then demonstrate what the craft will look like. It's a little bit abstract, and occasionally this can be difficult for people living with dementia if they do not understand what the final

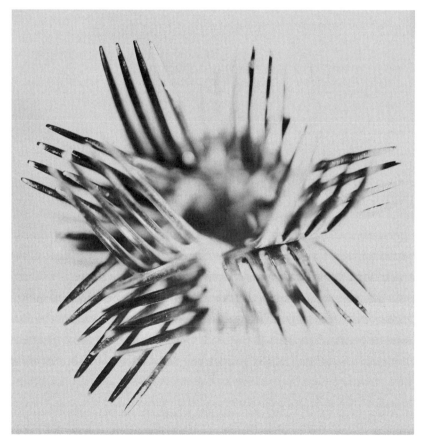

Figure 15.1. Using forks to make firework art is easy and fun, and it always looks great

product ought to look like. Then, step by step, encourage them to take the fork and dip it in paint. They can place the paint-dipped fork on the paper in whatever pattern they choose. Encourage and highlight every success, especially if they seem unsure at first.

Entertainment: Pre-Midnight Party

Many people living with dementia keep strange hours. Their internal clocks aren't working as well as they used to, so some people will be up all night while others just wake up every couple hours. Instead of trying to host a celebration at midnight, have it at noon! I have found that hosting activities and events before 2 pm is often the way to go: everyone feels more awake and engaged earlier in the day.

Food: New Year's Eve Fancy Cocktails/Mocktails

At your party, offer cocktails! Unless a doctor has provided permission for the individual living with dementia to consume alcohol, however, you may be relegated to serving only mocktails. If this is the case, there are many easy substitutes for actual liquor. Instead of filling champagne flutes with champagne, try using Sprite or another bubbly, clear soda.

Christmas

Craft: Popsicle Stick Christmas Trees

Easy and fun, popsicle stick Christmas trees make great ornaments (figure 15.2). Necessary items include popsicle sticks, paint, paper, buttons or small trinkets to decorate with, glue, and string. If asking clients to create the trees is going to be too difficult, given that it's a fairly abstract idea, make them ahead of time. Arrange popsicle sticks in triangle shapes and glue them together. Glue small strips of brown paper to the bottom popsicle stick to create a "trunk" for the tree. Get clients to help paint and decorate the trees and then tie string to them for easy hanging.

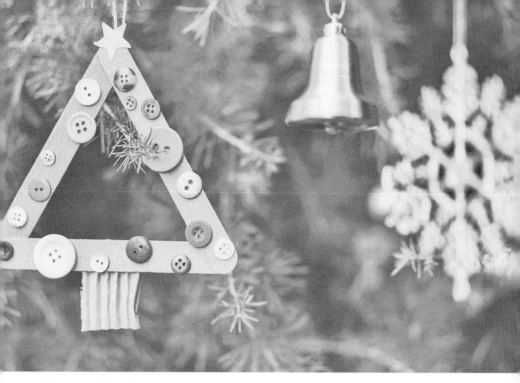

Figure 15.2. Popsicle sticks can be used to make Christmas tree ornaments

Entertainment: Bringing in Kids to Sing

Some of my most memorable moments working in residential dementia care are of those occasions when we brought in local preschool children to sing for our residents. The key to making this process run smoothly was to arrange the event with teachers at the school weeks in advance. Children coming to sing Christmas carols would come in the earlier part of the day and would arrive and leave within ninety minutes. Before the children left, some of them would walk around and hug my residents. I very clearly remember one of my residents, who was very advanced in her dementia, crying with joy as the children greeted her.

Food: Baking Cookies

Like they do on the Food Network when they're demonstrating a new recipe, I recommend having both a tray of prebaked cookies and a tray that you prepare with the person who has dementia. While one tray is in the oven, the other is already ready to be decorated. One of the biggest mistakes I made when I was first working with people who had dementia was allowing too much time to pass between events. There were a couple of times when I'd be working with my residents, happily baking and preparing something to eat, and then I'd lose half my group once the item went into the oven. In the twenty minutes that it took to bake the cookies, my residents would get distracted and bored.

Hanukkah

Craft: Watercolor Dreidels

Most craft stores offer wooden crafts to paint and decorate. For this particular craft, the only items you need are watercolor paint, paintbrushes, water, and wooden dreidels. (If you cannot find wooden dreidels, opt for printable paper options instead.) Ask the person with dementia "for help" painting the dreidels for decoration (figure 15.3). Suggesting that you are planning a party and need decor for the event is always a great way to get people engaged in assisting: you thereby create the impression that you need the craft to be done and that it isn't "just for fun."

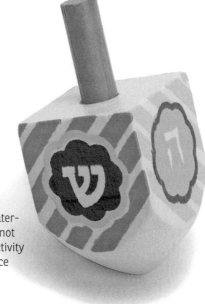

Figure 15.3. Painting watercolor dreidels provides not only an engaging art activity but also a fun game once the dreidels have dried

Entertainment: Dreidel-Spinning Game

There's almost nothing—in my opinion—that works as well for entertainment as competition-based games. Introduce the dreidel-spinning game to your client, loved one, or residents as a game that is best played with two or more people. Have them bet on which side the dreidel will land, and then whoever wins gets to take chips, coins, or candy from the other. Each person should start with a few chips that they are willing to bet in exchange for a dreidel roll. Any game that I've ever played with my clients with dementia that has been competition based has gone exceedingly well.

Food: Star of David Chocolate-Covered Pretzels

I found this tasty craft online and thought it was a perfect way to engage individuals living with dementia. Ingredients include stick pretzels, melted chocolate for dipping, and sprinkles for decoration. Start by melting chocolate in a bowl and laying out parchment paper on a table. Clients can dip the stick pretzels in chocolate and arrange them in a star shape on the parchment paper. Then allow these to dry and gently place in the refrigerator to solidify. If this is too challenging for your clients, you may want to make the shapes ahead of time and offer to let them decorate the stars.

Memorial Day / Veterans Day

Craft: Baskets for Local First Responders

One of my favorite crafts is basket creation for local first responders. This is a great craft for a holiday on which you are celebrating wartime heroes, local and abroad. Take basic laundry baskets and weave ribbon through the holes in the basket. Ribbons can be any color, but they make the most sense if they are those of the flag of the state or country you live in (figure 15.4). Fill the baskets with goodies and even make a day of it: bring the baskets to local law enforcement and other first responders. I remember vividly the day that we did this at my first

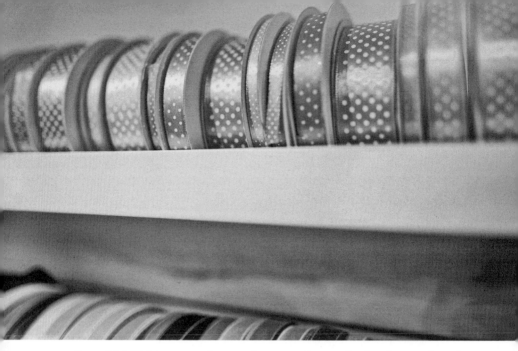

Figure 15.4. Ribbons are an inexpensive way to decorate baskets for a variety of occasions

senior living community: we rode our community's bus around town and stopped at the fire department and police station. The employees and volunteers at these places came onto our bus to accept their gifts, and my residents were overjoyed.

Entertainment: Veterans Celebration

Be sure to host or attend a celebration for local veterans. These are often very popular events inside of senior living communities, as many of the older adults who live there are veterans or know veterans. Veterans should receive mini flags and pins, along with a handshake from a local government official. When we hosted this type of event in senior housing, we'd bring in the city's first responders and local government to congratulate and shake hands with our vets. There were often a lot of smiles and joyful tears in the audience.

Food: Flag-Colored Parfaits

You can do this any time during the year, but I think it is especially important to celebrate your country's colors during a holiday when you're celebrating or remembering veterans. Parfaits are easy to make and fun to eat. Ingredients include Jell-O, pudding, and whipped cream. Make the Jell-O and pudding ahead of time and get help from the person with dementia you are working with to layer these items together in a parfait glass. (Clear glasses make the most sense so that everyone can see the colors.) Vanilla pudding can even be mixed with food coloring to match flag colors.

Thanksgiving

Craft: Name Cards

When I was younger, one of the more important things that my sister and I prepared each Thanksgiving were name cards for the table (figure 15.5). We very much enjoyed writing out each name place card, decorating it, and then putting it on the table in front of a plate. This craft is particularly good for people with dementia because it includes them in

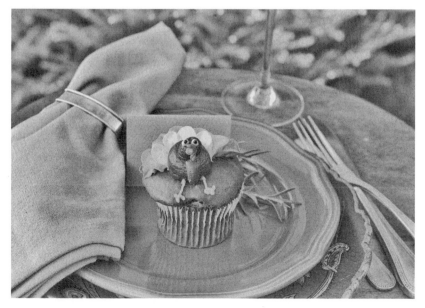

Figure 15.5. Making Thanksgiving name cards is a great way to include people living with dementia in the festivities

the festivities in a crucial way. Thanksgiving is, for most families, about bringing everyone together at one dinner table. Writing everyone's names is not only a good reminder of who is attending that evening, but it's also a way to help people with dementia feel involved. There are many crafts one might do with people with dementia that are not useful, but making name place cards is not one of them! They will definitely be used at dinner.

Entertainment: Planning a Parade Float
Watching the local, regional, or national parade live or on TV is an important Thanksgiving tradition for many people. A fun way to watch the parade in a more involved way—rather than just staring—is to brainstorm an imaginary float for the event. Grab a whiteboard or piece of paper and plan a float that you'll be making for the parade. It can be as detailed and creative as you want it to be. There are no wrong answers when it comes to making this parade float.

Food: Pumpkin Pie or Bread
The trick here, again, is to have a premade pie or bread and one that you'll be working on live. This allows everyone to eat and enjoy while the other one is in the oven baking. If pie is too hard to make, I recommend trying pumpkin bread instead.

CONCLUSION

There are so many ways to enjoy the holidays, and so many holidays to enjoy. These are just a few options for making the most of them. Crafts, baking, and events are best for people with dementia when they are kept fun and simple. Don't overthink it or worry too much that the activities will be too easy for them. It's better to have a craft that you need to add steps to than to have one that you need to simplify significantly for anyone to enjoy.

Hospice Activities

There are a number of misconceptions about hospice care and palliative care. One misconception is that hospice care and palliative care are the same thing. Another is that the patient in hospice care is too far gone to engage with others and enjoy activities. There's an assumption that once someone enters hospice care, that's the end of their life. I once heard someone say that hospice is just a way to "learn how to live differently," which was a really beautiful way to put it.

Palliative care is about providing relief for patients, usually from pain or a wound that won't heal. It does not mean that someone is dying, and some companies don't even offer both hospice and palliative care because they are very different services. Hospice care was created as a service—free for patients and their families through Medicare—to treat individuals whose conditions are worsening. "Worsening" does usually mean dying, but I've also seen many people "graduate" from hospice. If you graduate from hospice, this means that you've done so well in hospice care that you are no longer meeting the guidelines for receiving it. Another important aspect of hospice care is that it can be provided in senior living facilities, not just in homes.

"Rachael," Joe said as he appeared in my office door. "My dad is doing a lot better recently," he said gravely. I was confused. "That's . . . great, though, right?" I asked, unsure what Joe's feelings were on the subject.

"Of course," he said. "Yes, it's great, but . . . we love the hospice company you recommended. He's doing great and his pain is really manageable because of the extra care. I don't want them to bump him off of hospice care! What if he does so well that they take him off service? And then he gets worse again?" I shook my head. "Your dad is doing really well on hospice, you're right," I replied. "But he's still declining enough that they'll keep him on. They just downgraded his diet to mechanical soft, and, in my experience, diet downgrades usually count as a reason to keep someone on hospice."

Joe nodded slowly. "All right," he said. "I hope so. My dad is doing better because of that extra attention. And he really, really loves that hospice volunteer who comes in and plays music for him!"

Joe's father stayed on hospice for another month before passing away quietly in his room. Joe met me in the hallway the day after his dad died, smiling through his tears. "Thank you for your help. I know my dad lived out the rest of his days pain-free and pleasantly because of hospice."

My experience is that, when most people hear the word "hospice," they panic. I've watched families fight it, tooth and nail, trying not to put their loved ones on hospice, saying that it's not time yet. Often, they are wrong: it is time, but the fear is that hospice will hasten death. One thing that is true about hospice is that they do stop taking measures to prolong life; for example, a patient on hospice has to do what's called "revoking hospice" in order to go to the hospital. This means that their family is choosing to send them to the hospital—therefore invoking life-saving measures—so they have to give up hospice care. The patient can usually get back on hospice services after they return from the hospital, but it takes time and paperwork.

The goal of hospice is to provide extra care and resources for both the patient and the patient's family during a time of progressive decline in health. My own grandmother used hospice for almost a year. She lost her two-year battle with brain cancer when I was eighteen, but her decline and my family's subsequent suffering was made significantly more bearable with the aid of hospice. Hospice offered counseling and support groups, and my grandmother was provided a music therapist who came in to sing for her. Although it means that a person has to admit that there is a decline in their loved one's condition, inviting hospice into the home or senior living community can provide significant relief.

Many hospice companies have volunteers that work with them regularly. These volunteers often provide services such as music therapy, art therapy, or pet therapy for the patients on hospice. Hospice organizations recognize the importance of engagement even during someone's decline. Don't be afraid to ask the hospice company you are working with about activities and engagement for your loved one.

MUSIC THERAPY

Music is perhaps one of the most powerful ways to connect with others (figure 16.1). Even in late stages of dementia, music can have a positive impact on alertness, engagement, and happiness. Hsin Hua Chu and colleagues (2014) studied the effectiveness of music therapy on depression and dementia and found that group music therapy decreased depression in adults with dementia. While the group setting was the focus of their research, countless other studies have found that even individualized music sessions prove to be positive in working with people who have dementia. If your loved one's experiences with music are better when they are shared, however, then having a music therapist or family member in the room during the session could be beneficial. Music sessions go most smoothly when the client's family knows what type of music their loved one enjoys because then no time is wasted trying to find out what pleases the person the music is being played for.

Whenever one of my residents or clients was actively dying, whether they were on hospice or not, I'd bring a music player into their room and set up their favorite tunes. I could not always tell if they were paying

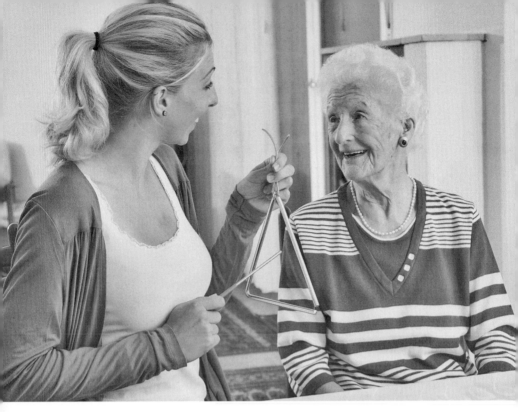

Figure 16.1. Music therapy can positively impact alertness, engagement, and happiness, even in the late stages of dementia

attention to it directly, but I noted that people's expressions seemed to soften when the music started playing. Even if someone's eyes were closed and they weren't acknowledging anyone, it did feel like the music made a difference. I made bringing music into someone's room and leaving it on a regular practice of mine. Often, clients' families appreciated this small gesture.

PET THERAPY

At this point, Millie spent most of her day in her room. She was hallucinating, which meant that she was often seeing or hearing things that weren't there. Often, what she heard was people talking, so real human beings coming into her room on top of that tired her out. One of the only things that did work for Millie was pet therapy.

The assisted living building where I worked had a couple of hospice companies that they regularly paired with. My favorite hospice company had anywhere from one to six of our residents on their caseload. They were so gracious that when they brought dogs, cats, or bunnies in for their own clients, they would also bring the animals around to the rest of my residents (figure 16.2).

It was almost hard to notice how advanced Millie's dementia was when she was petting the large, furry dog that came by once a week. Normally, Millie would spend her mornings getting angry with the people who came in her room (some real, some not) but her frustration ceased immediately upon the dog's entrance.

As you may already be aware, animals can be extremely therapeutic. Many hospice organizations offer pet therapy, and these pets are certified and trained. They are safe to be in homes or in senior living buildings, trained not to eat anything off the floor, and taught to be

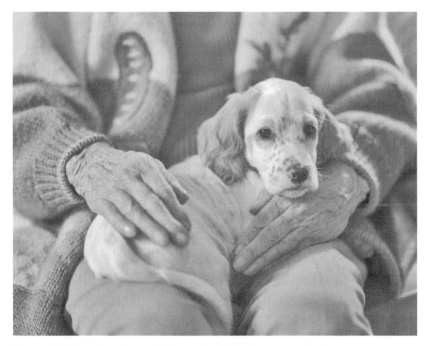

Figure 16.2. Spending time with live animals can be extremely therapeutic

careful around walkers and wheelchairs. When someone is bedbound or stays mostly in their room, bringing the engagement to them may be the best option. Even if someone cannot speak or sit up, they can still stroke soft fur.

ART THERAPY

Even when someone can't get out of bed, they can still participate in art activities (figure 16.3). They can look through a book of classic art pieces, or maybe they can even paint or draw. Whether the hospice company offers this or not, it is easy to engage someone in art—particularly if they used to be an artist or enjoyed looking at art. Bring in ceramics or other pieces that have a unique feel and then ask the person with dementia to "feel" the difference and explain it to you. Another great option is aquapaints, made by a company called Active Minds.

Figure 16.3. Art therapy can include making or looking at art and can be done in a range of settings

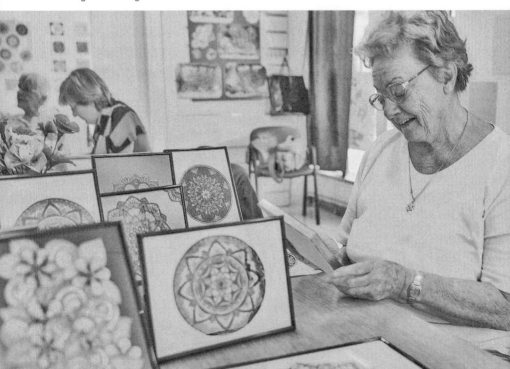

Aquapaints require only a paintbrush and a cup of water; images appear on the paper as the person brushes water over it, and so it is a virtually mess-free activity. When the aquapaints paper dries, it becomes blank again and so can be painted over and over.

WEIGHTED OR ACTIVITY BLANKETS

There's a lot of evidence that weighted blankets provide comfort to people—and not just those with dementia. The blankets make people feel like they're being hugged, more technically described as deep-pressure stimulation. Such stimulation causes the brain to release serotonin, helping people relax and feel less anxious even after only five minutes (Mullen, Champagne, Krishnamurty, Dickson, & Gao, 2008).Weighted blankets are often offered by hospice companies, along with activity blankets (figure 16.4). Activity blankets are often handmade blankets with small activities sewn onto them. These activities range from strings

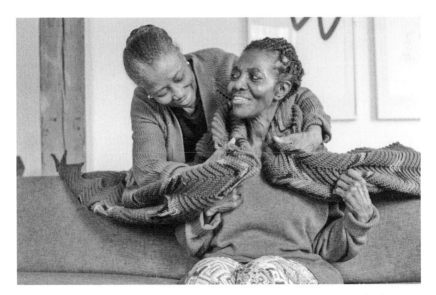

Figure 16.4. Activity and weighted blankets can provide stimulation and relaxation

to braid together all the way to finger puppets. Put simply, they are items to tinker with and touch. For people in very advanced stages of dementia, these blankets can provide relief for restless, anxious hands. You may notice that many people in later stages of dementia are often touching or reaching for things but then seem unsure about what exactly they want. These blankets are designed to engage someone right in their own lap. I do, however, want to discourage heated blankets, just because these can malfunction or become dangerous if left unwatched.

HAND MASSAGE AND NAIL CARE

Touch and positive dementia caregiving go hand in hand, pun intended. When working with people who have dementia, I have found that positive touch goes a long way. Hand massage and/or nail care can also encourage conversation, even if that conversation is mostly one-sided (figure 16.5). I personally have had full-out conversations with people

Figure 16.5. Hand massage, and other positive touch, such as nail care, can encourage conversation

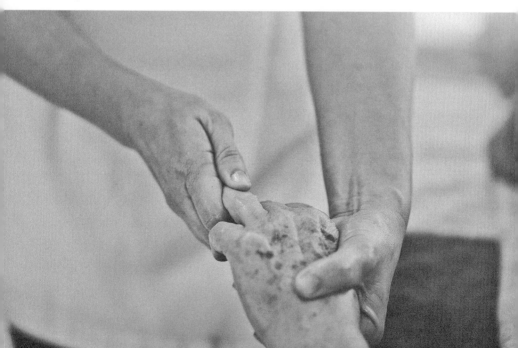

who can't speak, especially while helping them with their nails. Almost everyone loves a little extra attention, and extended hand-to-hand contact can be really positive.

A special note: some senior living companies consider trimming someone's nails to be a medical procedure, which means that the employees who perform the nail care must be nurses or another type of medical practitioner. While anyone can paint another person's nails, not everyone can trim or cut them.

FOLDING AND SORTING

Jerry hummed to himself as he folded hand towels (figure 16.6). Normally, Jerry was anxious and always trying to get out of his La-Z-Boy chair to head out the door. Unfortunately for Jerry, this was not a safe option: his dementia had progressed significantly in the months prior. His reasons for wanting to leave the house were important to him, for he felt that his son needed to see him. He also believed that his son, now 55, was only 15. Folding distracted him from his near-constant worry about his son.

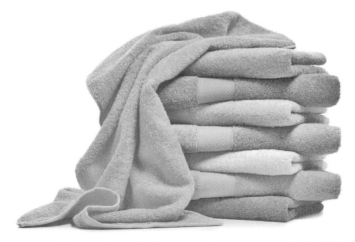

Figure 16.6. Folding towels, and other appropriate chores, makes individuals living with dementia feel helpful, which can brighten their spirits

His hospice company had also found that asking Jerry to help clean the windows kept him occupied. They'd hand him a rag, spritz the window with cleaning solution, and try to talk to him about something other than his son. Even if only for fifteen minutes, it worked. That was fifteen minutes during which he was calm and content.

Chores, as we have seen, are excellent activities for people living with dementia. They make individuals feel useful and helpful, which in turn brightens spirits and souls.

CONCLUSION

All of these options are great for individuals who are bedbound or whose ability to move is limited. Of course, not everyone on hospice or in need of hospice care is bedbound or limited in their ability to move. It is best to continue to encourage as much activity as possible for as long as possible. While you don't want to exhaust or overwhelm someone with dementia, suddenly ceasing activity because they can do less is not a good option. It is always best to simplify activities rather than take them away. For example, if someone can no longer fold towels at the same speed that they used to or if they get "stuck" often, hand them one towel at a time. You aren't taking the activity away: you are just modifying it to meet their ability.

17

Meals and Baking

We don't normally think of meals as activities or as ways to engage people living with dementia. We think of meals as a means to an end: the goal is to get the person seated, make sure they eat and drink, and then move on with the day. This is true for caregivers in both community living settings and home care settings. While there is a difference between a sit-down meal and a baking activity, the point should be the same: to engage the person living with dementia and facilitate a sense of autonomy and independence. How do we accomplish this, especially when many people with cognitive impairments have trouble eating and drinking independently? How do we help people with dementia feel as though they are making choices regarding their meals, even if they are preplanned for them?

It is quite possible to turn a meal into an activity in and of itself. In this chapter, we review some ways to get people with dementia to eat and drink more at meal times as well as baking and cooking recipes that you and the person or persons with dementia can work on together.

THE IMPORTANCE OF SNACKS

Caroline was distraught, to say the least. Right around 6:30 pm every day, she'd come out of her room, crying and yelling for her parents. It was truly heart wrenching to hear Caroline's cries. "Momma! Daddy! Please, where are you?" she'd yell while wheeling her wheelchair down the hallway. The interesting thing was this: Caroline was never, ever like this during the day. In fact, she was downright calm and collected the majority of the time. Caroline had a really bad case of sundowning—a syndrome where people with cognitive impairments get more agitated later in the day—and this resulted in her cries for help. At a certain point, I ran out of ideas as to how to comfort her. I had tried talking to her, holding her hand, and seeing if she needed to use the restroom. With nothing obvious left to try, I happened to catch sight of some chocolate pudding cups that were left over from a previous activity. I grabbed a spoon and a pudding cup and walked it over to Caroline. As I reached out to hand it to her, she stopped mid-yell. "Momma, where are—oh! Thank you for this," she said, smiling calmly and accepting the snack. I was relieved, but also amazed: Caroline was just hungry. She was not able to tell us that, and so instead, her hunger revealed itself through sadness and confusion.

Providing food and drinks throughout the day is imperative in dementia care. Often, people living with dementia are unable to tell us what their basic needs are. Because they may not be able to tell us verbally, they may act out in unexpected ways. Think about how many times you take a drink of water throughout the day: do you think that someone with dementia can remember to grab a glass of water that often? Generally, the answer is no. It's up to the caregiver to provide water and snacks between meals, even if the person with dementia isn't asking for them. Urinary tract infections (UTIs) are rampant in senior living, especially among older women with dementia. There are a few reasons for this uptick in UTIs, but one of them is not taking in enough fluids, a problem that can be easily addressed by providing more water throughout the day. Many people with dementia don't drink enough water, and this can deeply affect the way their bodies function.

Turning snack time into an activity is a great way to encourage eating and drinking, as is baking, cooking, or hosting a themed party.

SETTING THE SCENE

The goal of setting the scene is to encourage people with dementia to eat and drink more. When you are preparing for a meal or baking activity, there are a few steps you should take before beginning. Some of these may seem obvious, but they are all necessary. No matter if this is an individual activity or a group one, the gist will be very similar.

1. Ensure that the individual washes their hands. If they are unable to wash their hands with ease, wet a washcloth with warm water and soap and wash their hands for them. Most people are familiar with the idea of washing up before a meal, and adding this into your routine will encourage the person you're caring for to eat more. It feels normal to start a meal with clean hands, and a sense of normalcy should be maintained, even in advanced stages of dementia.

2. Start the meal by playing music in the background. Music without lyrics tends to be the best bet, as some people will begin singing along and lose focus on the meal itself.

3. Remove distractions such as baby dolls or television. Many people who believe that the baby dolls are real will try to feed the baby instead of feeding themselves. If this is the case, suggest that the "baby needs a nap" while the meal is going on.

4. Ensure that there is a difference between the color of the plate and the color of the food on the plate. It can be difficult for people with dementia to discriminate between colors that look too similar. Brightly colored plates are best for encouraging

eating. There's also some research that suggests that if you use brightly colored glasses rather than clear, people with dementia will even drink more (Kingston, 2017). In both cases, bright colors in food service ware are easier for people with dementia to see and help them stay focused on the activity.

5. Ask "Would you like this or this?" instead of "Are you hungry?" Providing two options allows the person with dementia to make a decision, but it is a decision between one of just two possibilities. You are much more likely to get a no or "I'm not hungry" when the question is open ended. Showing the two options—holding up a cereal box in one hand and an oatmeal box in the other, for example—is a great way to visually display what you are talking about. Even people who have trouble communicating can point to which food they'd like to eat.

6. When you are planning something like a baking activity, it's important to pick a time of day at which the person or persons you are caring for will be interested in eating. For example, planning to make pudding at 9:00 am will probably not elicit the same positive response as making it right before lunch or as mid-afternoon snack.

7. When it comes to water, provide it without asking. Asking "Are you thirsty?" or "Do you want a drink?" may get a no even when that person needs water.

8. You may need to adjust the activity or meal when utensils become a problem. Many people in more advanced stages of dementia have trouble using utensils to eat or to prepare food with.

IN A COMMUNITY SETTING

The staff had gathered everyone in the dining room for dinner except Townsend. Townsend was agitated, as she often was later in the day, and she became ever more agitated if she had to wait for her meal to be served. Although it would have been potentially easier to serve Townsend her meal in another room, the staff was shorthanded. There was no way for staff to watch her for choking and keep serving the other residents. So instead of bringing Townsend in at the same time as everyone else, they waited until everyone was seated and soups were passed out. Then one of the staff members went to fetch Townsend. She was able to get seated and be served immediately, which calmed her down significantly. She did not like waiting more than a minute to get her soup, so this approach worked well.

In a community setting, the goal is always to get as many people as possible engaged at one time. When it comes to meals, this can be a real challenge. When it comes to a baking or cooking activity, it can also be a real challenge. A best practice is to plan ahead, decide who will be attending the activity, and then try to get everyone in the activity space at one time. If that doesn't work, engage the ones who are sitting there with a small task while you gather the rest of the group. Put on some music and keep everyone in the room occupied while you work to get the group together.

Diet restrictions may pose a challenge when you are working with a group. If a resident is unable to chew or swallow well, they may have been switched to a puree or mechanical soft diet. Keep this in mind as you are planning your baking activity, and gather a group who can enjoy each step of the process. Remember that telling someone with dementia "not to eat that" may not work. They may still reach out and take the food item without realizing that they cannot swallow it properly.

If you don't want to change the particular activity, put different residents at different stations. For example, if you are making chocolate pudding and cookie cups, but Heather can't chew cookies, seat her at a table away from the cookies where she can stir the pudding mix.

The best activities are always ones where the bulk of the work is done before the residents get started. An activity can quickly go off the rails if there is too much time spent prepping or waiting for the item to bake. Baking activities are best if there is minimal stove or oven time: the less waiting before enjoying, the better.

AT HOME

"I already ate breakfast," Aaron protested when his caregiver put a plate of waffles in front of him. "I had cereal," he said, pushing the plate away. Aaron had not in reality eaten breakfast that day. His caregiver knew better than to argue, however. "Oh, I know," Stu said. "I just made some waffles for myself and wanted your opinion. Can you taste some and let me know if they're any good?" Aaron nodded, happy to be asked for his opinion on the matter. Ten minutes later, Aaron's plate was clean, and he'd forgotten about the cereal he believed that he'd already eaten. "Breakfast was great," he said, smiling.

Aaron's caregiver knew better than to ask if Aaron was hungry. The same thing applies when preparing a baking or cooking activity. Instead of asking the people you are caring for if they want to bake cookies, the best approach is to say, "I'm going to bake cookies. Can you help me?" You are stating your intention—baking cookies—and then asking them for their help. Most people will say yes when asked for assistance.

When it's only one person, a great strategy is to have two choices planned out ahead of time. "Would you like to bake chocolate chip cookies, or would you prefer muffins?" allows the individual to make a choice but still choose one of the preplanned options. This doesn't work as well in a group, since everyone will have different opinions on what to make.

Get the activity started as soon as their hands are washed. People living with dementia, especially those in moderate or advanced stages, do not always have much patience. They may get up and walk away if they aren't immediately engaged in an activity. If you need to use the oven, preheat it ahead of time. Plan an activity to do while you wait for the baking to finish.

CREATIVE ACTIVITIES

Taste Testing

Taste testing is exactly what it sounds like: get some different types of cookies, for example, and have them taste test each one (figure 17.1). This is a simple activity that involves zero baking and very minimal preparation. Bring in a whiteboard and write their opinions about each cookie on the board; this helps everyone feel like their opinion is valuable.

Figure 17.1. Taste testing is a simple activity that helps everyone feel like their opinion is valuable

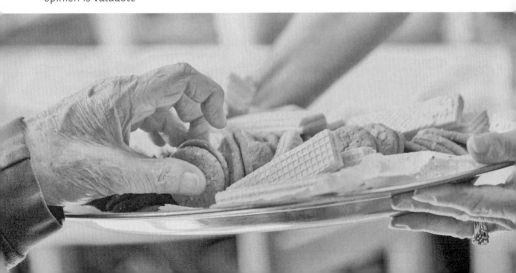

Mixed-Drinks Party

Although occasionally someone with dementia has a doctor's order to drink alcoholic drinks (it's true!) usually it is not advisable to provide alcohol to a person with dementia without a doctor's previous permission. It could interact poorly with certain medications, or it could cause more confusion. In any case, it is possible to have a "mixed drink" without any added alcohol (figure 17.2). Host a gathering where the drinks are all a mix of different juices and flavors and are served in fun, colorful cups. Have your residents, clients, or loved ones make the beverages with you. You can also provide the drinks for the party, premade, and have everyone taste test different drinks.

Figure 17.2. Mixed drinks can be made with a variety of different juices and flavors, without any added alcohol

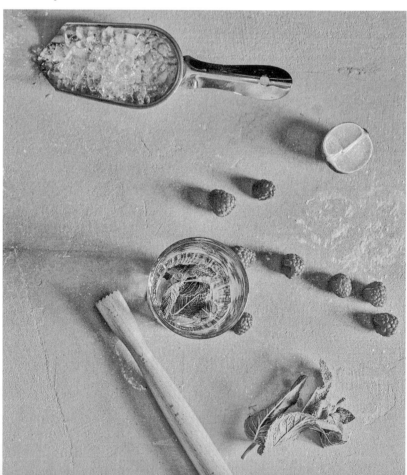

Dirt Cups

Most people know what a "dirt cup" is, although there are a few different variations on the same recipe (figure 17.3). Break it down into steps for the person or people you are working with. If this is a group activity, have different residents complete different tasks.

The ingredients you need are instant pudding mix, milk, cookies, measuring cups, plastic bags, spoons, and cups. A best practice is to mix some pudding ahead of time and put it in the fridge. This way, when you start, you will already have some pudding to work with. Have the people you are working with spoon pudding into each cup. Put the cookies in plastic bags and let each person crush their own cookies with their hands or by hitting the bags (tightly sealed) on the table. Once they have crushed the cookies, have them sprinkle the cookie pieces out on top of the pudding cups.

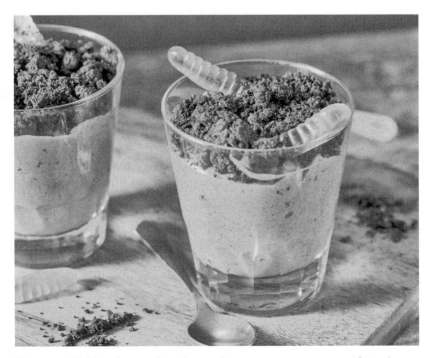

Figure 17.3. Making dirt cups is an interactive way to engage a group of people

Soft Pretzels

Have your client or residents create their own soft pretzels (figure 17.4). Recipes vary, so find one that you like! Make the dough ahead of time. Have your residents or client twist the pretzels and then have them dip the pretzels in the egg mixture before they place them on a baking sheet. They can sprinkle each one with salt before you put the tray into the oven.

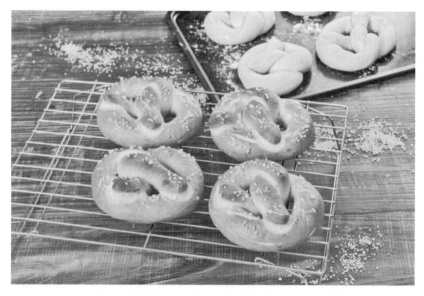

Figure 17.4. When making soft pretzels, it's best to make the dough ahead of time, but allow the person with dementia to twist their own pretzel

Cookie Bake and Decoration

These are great for any time of year, and can be adjusted accordingly. No matter the holiday, find cookie-cutters and toppers that match. The ingredients for this activity are premade cookies, cookie mix, measuring cups and spoons, mixing spoons, cookie sheets, cooking spray, sprinkles, and decorating gel. If baking cookies ahead of time is too much work, buy premade cookies to decorate (figure 17.5). No matter

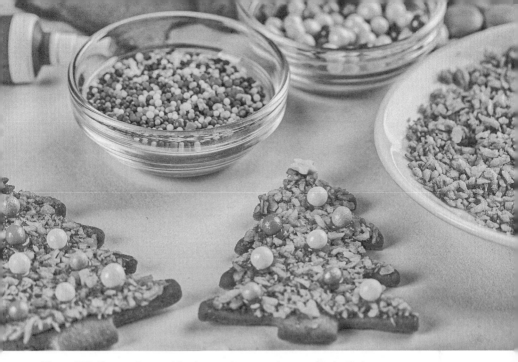

Figure 17.5. Decorating cookies lets each person be creative in their own way

what, have cookies available to decorate while the one batch is baking. The goal, as always, is to keep the person or people engaged throughout the whole process to decrease the chance of anyone wandering off. The best thing about this particular activity is that each person gets to be creative on their cookies—and then eat what they made.

Birthday Cupcakes

I love activities that have a distinct purpose or holiday affiliation. Celebrate individual or group birthdays with this activity, which is much like the cookie decorating activity (figure 17.6). You'll need cupcake papers, a cupcake pan, cake mix, measuring cups and spoons, decorating utensils, and gels/sprinkles. If baking cupcakes is too much work, buy or make cupcakes ahead of time. Break the cupcake baking or decorating down into easy steps by providing one item at a time, or, if you have a group of residents, by giving each small group a task. For example, one group can work on stirring the batter while the other lays the cupcake papers into the cupcake pan.

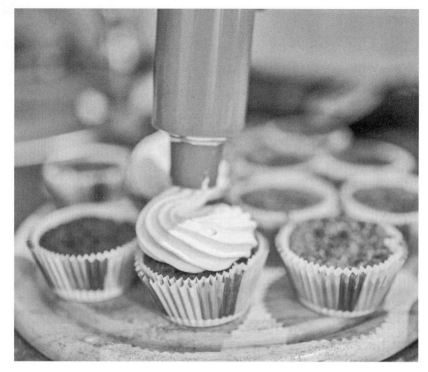

Figure 17.6. Baking and decorating cupcakes is a great way to celebrate individual and group birthdays

Pancakes, Quesadillas, Grilled Cheese, and More

Don't be afraid of a little open flame! Plenty of people with dementia can still handle turning items over on a stovetop. We never want to take tasks away from people while they can still do them. Start a stovetop-based activity with a few safety precautions in place, and you will have a successful activity (figure 17.7). Choose what you want to make and then ensure that there is plenty of room at the stove. Have a chair or two nearby in case someone wants to sit down. Make sure, of course, that the person with dementia is not so advanced that they are unsure of how a stovetop works, and let everyone know that it can be very hot. This type of activity, since it does involve some minimal risk, is best for someone in an early or early-middle stage of dementia.

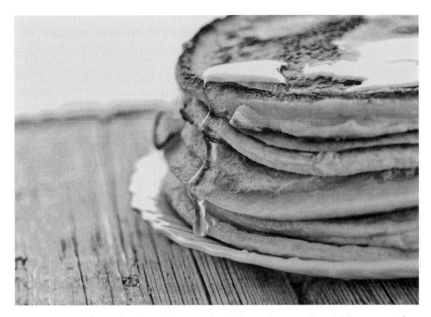

Figure 17.7. Don't be afraid to allow people in the early or early-middle stages of dementia to help with stovetop cooking, such as making pancakes

No-Bake Items

Any large grocery store will have a collection of no-bake items. Even treats like pie often have a no-bake option, where the pie is made entirely with pudding and finished in the fridge or freezer. If you are short on time or find other items on this list too difficult but still want to try a baking activity, this may be the one to attempt. It requires minimal work, but it can be stretched out into a larger, longer activity if more people are involved.

18

Brain Exercise

Clive did not really speak much at all. He was a retired pastor and had a PhD in theology and often perked up at the sound of religious songs coming through our music player. Occasionally you would hear a few words from Clive, usually in response to food or music. "This is good," he offered one day at lunch. Clive's family visited often but usually didn't know what to say to him. "He doesn't really talk anymore," his wife said, sighing.

One of my favorite things to do with my residents was a fill-in-the-blank activity. I had a book full of lyrics and short words of advice; I would read the first part of a song line or aphorism and my residents would fill in the rest. "A rolling stone . . . ," I would start. "Gathers no moss!" they'd call back. I remember Clive sitting in the back of the room, quiet as usual. His head was down and he appeared to be sleeping peacefully, ignoring the exclamations around them. I came to a couple of Bible verses and hesitated: I did not like bringing religion into a group if I wasn't sure what religion each person was. I shrugged to myself, figuring I would give it a try.

"And if a house be divided against itself . . . ," I started. A voice, normally soft and hesitant, sounded from the back. "That house cannot stand: Mark 3:25," Clive called. "Whoa!" one of the care assistants said, whirling around. "Was that Clive?" We looked over at him to see a small smile cross his face.

Brain exercises come in many shapes and forms. For all of my time working in dementia care, I am still happily shocked when a person with aphasia (a disorder characterized by speech-related challenges) answers a riddle, rhyme, or lyric. It never fails to amaze me that despite someone's inability to speak, they can still sing or recite a common phrase.

There is a lot of anecdotal evidence suggesting that music and rhythm are left mostly unscathed by dementia, but research has yet to explain just why there is this almost "awakening" for some people with dementia when they are exposed to music. Other activities like puzzles and trivia questions are great ways to make your brain work in a way that it doesn't normally. Anytime the brain is engaged in a new task, it must engage in new cognitive processes. This promotes the creation of new connections between neurons and sometimes the development of new brain cells (La Rue, 2010). Because dementia damages the brain, these new neurons and connections help reduce the speed at which cognitive decline occurs. Think of it this way: the more neural connections and neurons you have, the longer it's going to take for damage in the brain to affect them all. A *cognitive reserve* has been created. Thus while they are not able to cure dementia, these brain exercises may slow down the deterioration. From people with mild cognitive impairment all the way to individuals with severe dementia, brain exercise is an important part of every day.

Christine had a diagnosis of mild cognitive impairment, which meant that, while she was aware of—and annoyed by—her condition, it did not prevent her from living alone and going about her business. Still, she wanted to see if she could improve her current condition by strengthening her brain. Christine found a website that was proven to help individuals improve their memories and reaction times. She dedicated herself to working on it once a day for a week. After a month of doing this, Christine began to feel like she'd improved: her memory seemed better, or, at least, she felt more successful and happy. Christine added some extra exercise to her day and also added a weekly Scrabble date with a friend. She kept a three-hundred-piece puzzle out on her dining room table that she'd work on when she walked into the room. Slowly, piece by piece, it came together. While years ago she may have thought of these kinds of activities as frivolous or just games, now they felt crucial to her daily routine.

When making a daily plan for my residents or clients, I include at least one cognitive exercise. A cognitive exercise can be anything that makes someone focus, learn, or push beyond their own limitations.

CROSSWORDS AND PUZZLES

You are going to want to find a crossword puzzle or jigsaw puzzle that fits the cognitive level of the person you are working with (figure 18.1). For example, a three-hundred-piece puzzle for someone with a moderate degree of dementia is going to be much too challenging. There is a certain level of frustration that we want the person to experience, so the puzzle you pick should not be easy, but it also should not be devastatingly difficult for them to complete. We do not want them feeling like they're incapable or dumb. I like large-print crossword puzzles that are easy to see and write on. I also like jigsaw puzzles with large pieces that are easy to pick up. The key, though, is to find a puzzle that isn't made specifically for children; for example, you would not want to buy a puzzle of cartoon princesses. Floor puzzles often contain fewer pieces, and the individual pieces are bigger.

There are a couple ways to successfully introduce puzzles. I have seen it go well when the puzzle is left out on the table for a person with dementia to "find." Most times, though, the puzzle is more success-

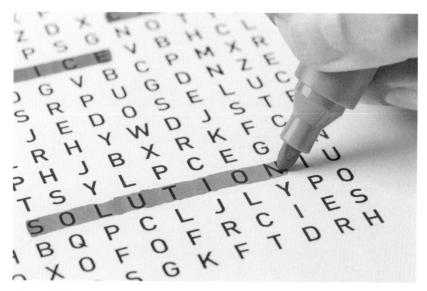

Figure 18.1. Word search puzzles challenge people living with dementia, without making them feel incapable or dumb

ful when introduced directly. Saying something like "Can you help me with this puzzle? I'm having some difficulty" is a great introduction. This makes the person feel important and needed. It also makes them feel as though it is okay to struggle, because you have admitted to struggling.

FINISHING LYRICS AND LINES

You read the first part of a lyric, common saying, or pieces of advice that everyone has heard, and the people you are working with fill in the blank. This is my favorite thing to do with people living with dementia. It's my favorite thing because it can be used in almost any situation. I have seen this game work wonders in individuals with mild cognitive impairment as well as individuals with advanced Alzheimer disease. "I can't believe I know these," I've often heard people say, laughing joyfully. People with dementia remember lyrics and common phrases even when they cannot remember what they ate for breakfast. It is also common for individuals who have trouble speaking to be able to finish the sayings as well. I have learned not to underestimate anyone with dementia when playing this game, so just go for it, see how it goes, and adjust accordingly. For example, if the person you are working with is great with naming famous song lyrics, find as many lyrics as you can. Make them feel as successful as possible.

These are great to do one-on-one or with a big group. If you are gathering a group, get everyone in a circle around you and be sure to speak loudly. The key here is to enunciate as best you can, even when working with one individual. When I do this activity—which is often— I start with an example. Saying "I will say the first part, and you say the second part" helps set the scene. "For example, if I say, 'A rolling stone,' you would say, 'gathers no moss.'" Sometimes, this game needs no introduction. You may be surprised at how quickly the person or people you are playing with catch on. I keep track of which lines go best, and I start with those. It is easier for people to catch on when they understand the rules of the game immediately.

IMPROVISATION GAMES

Improvisation is a type of theater where participants make stories and plays up on the spot. Nearly nothing is planned ahead of time, and while there are a few "rules" of improv, there are not many constraints. I myself have been performing improv comedy for nearly a decade, and I find that a lot of the skills I use on stage are great brain workouts (figure 18.2). I began using short improv games and exercises with my mild cognitive impairment group with much success.

Zip, Zap, Zop: One person starts, points to another person in the group, and says "zip." The person who gets pointed to then points to another person and says "zap." That person points to another and says "zop." Then it's back to "zip," and it continues from there. If the group is

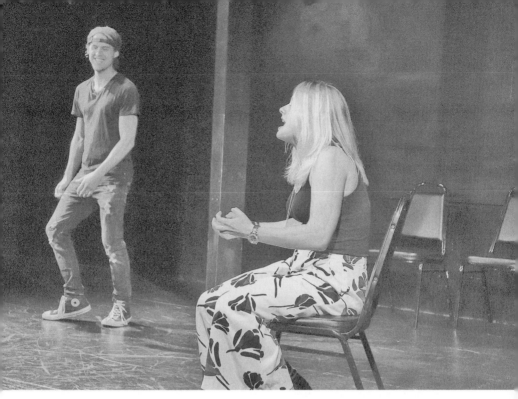

Figure 18.2. There are a number of improvisation games that people with dementia can play that act as great brain workouts. Used with permission of Steel City Improv Theater in Pittsburgh, PA.

getting too good at it, add other words, like "lip, lap, lop." If the group is having trouble, write the words up on a whiteboard.

Clap, Clap: Try to clap at the same exact time as another person. It should make one, single sound. The person who receives the clap then turns to another and tries to clap at the same time as them. It's fun and a good game for attention and focus.

Dave Delivers Donuts in Denver: Pick a letter of the alphabet and name a person's name that starts with that letter. The next person names an action or object that starts with that letter. The third person says a place that starts with that letter. Then, you all say the sentence together.

Group Imagination: Tell a story together. The leader facilitates the story and asks each person to add details to it. For example, say "Let's pretend this is a dentist's office. What color is on the walls in the waiting room?" You may be surprised by how vivid the group's imagination is!

Group Rhyme or Association: Name an object and have the person to your left name something that rhymes with it or, alternatively, something it makes them think of. The person to their left names a word that rhymes with the word they just heard and so forth.

Red Ball: You have an invisible ball that you call "red ball." Take red ball and throw it to someone, saying, "Red ball" when you throw it. When they catch the ball, they say, "Red ball," and when they throw it, they say it again. If the group does too well with this, add a green ball that gets tossed at the same time as the red ball.

These activities work best with groups of three to eight people, although they can be modified for one-on-one or pairs. Suggest that you are going to be doing a fun brain exercise and explain the rules. You will have to modify the game or switch to a new one if people are having a hard time with it. As always, the goal is to ensure that people feel challenged but successful. These games work best with higher-functioning individuals but can be modified to meet the needs of people in more moderate stages of dementia.

BRAINSTORMING

All this activity really needs is a whiteboard and whiteboard marker (figure 18.3). You are going to name something, such as a holiday that is coming up, and talk about it with the group. A great example is, "What kinds of foods do you eat at Christmas or Hanukkah?" The group calls out things that they eat during the holidays, and you write each one on the whiteboard so that they can see their suggestion written down. Pause to talk about each example, and allow for plenty of stories and discussion.

This activity works well one-on-one or with a group. Start by saying that you will be working together to come up with a list, but that you do not want to repeat suggestions. Write each one down on the board, and circle it if it comes up a couple times.

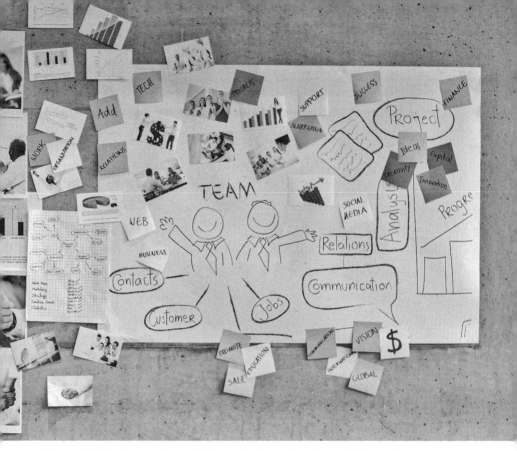

Figure 18.3. Brainstorming activities can help spark stories and discussions

WORD WALL

A whiteboard or a chalkboard works well for this activity. You will be asking the person or people living with dementia to name words that start with certain letters, include certain letters, or make them think of words that are already up on the board. In this particular photo, we have a wall with magnetic letters.

Ask the people you are working with to help you come up with words to add to the board. If you put up a letter, such as "P," ask them to tell you some words that start with the letter P. If that's too easy, put up a few letters on the board, such as "P, A, E, L, T, M." The group should name words that include the letter "P" but can include as many or as few of the other letters as possible.

CONCLUSION

Brain exercise is an important part of everyday life for most everyone, particularly people living with cognitive impairments. When we encourage mental exercise, we also encourage individuals to get active, improve their moods, and strengthen their bonds with one another. Deciding that "they can't do this type of thing anymore" before trying it is an incredibly dangerous path to start down. The worst thing that would happen is that you need to switch or modify the activity.

Artwork and Creativity

Dani had been an artist her whole life. She had worked often on canvas with colored pencils and acrylic paint. She raised a couple of kids, and while her husband was the main provider, she had earned some regular income with her art. Now that she had dementia, Dani still described herself as an artist, but she didn't paint much anymore. In fact, her daughter, Kara, told everyone that she couldn't paint. "Eh, Mom really can't paint anymore," she said. "I've asked her if she wants to try, but she just says she'd rather do something else . . . so, I don't push it." Finally, with some teaching and coaxing, Kara decided to try again. Instead of asking if Dani wanted to paint, her daughter set up a canvas and some paintbrushes near her mother's spot at the table. When Dani came down for lunch, she sat in front of the paint. "What do you want me to do with this?" Dani asked, sighing loudly. "I need more art for the new house," Kara explained. "Paint that tree across the yard there," she said, pointing out the window. Dani shrugged and began to paint. An hour passed, and Dani continued to paint. Finally, she was done. There on the canvas stood a beautiful, intricate, textured tree with a blue-gray sky behind it.

People living with dementia do not quickly lose their ability to create music or art. Often, they just need a little bit of coaxing or a slightly modified activity to get started. Instead of asking her mother what she wanted to do, Kara told Dani what she needed. Once Dani got started, her love of painting was revived and her long experience guided her anew. I have often found that watching someone with dementia do something they love is to watch their cognitive impairments fade, if only for a few minutes.

In this chapter, we go through some arts and crafts activities that work well for people with dementia. These can be done in residential settings or at home. Studies have shown that when caregivers and their care receivers with dementia work together on creative art projects, caregivers develop an increased awareness and understanding of their loved ones, as well as discovering an enjoyable activity that they can share (Mondro, Connell, Li, & Reed, 2018).

First, here are rules to live by when choosing a craft for a person with dementia:

- Ensure that it is not too challenging. Typically, anything more than two steps is too hard. If they have to choose the paint, open it themselves, set the canvas up, arrange the flowers they need to paint a picture of, and then paint that picture, that is too many steps.

- Choose a craft that is not too abstract. For example, a craft designed for a child such as fashioning a paper plate to look like a spider (hanging strings from the plate for legs, painting it, etc.) is typically too abstract and confusing for someone living with dementia. You will hear questions like "Why are we doing this?" and "What is this supposed to be, again?"

- Ensure that the craft you are choosing is not childish. While it can be a craft that you borrowed and adapted from a children's craft, it should not be childlike. Many people with dementia do not like coloring because they regard it as something kids do, not adults.

- Pick a craft and then lay out all the materials ahead of time. No matter whether you are working with a group of residents or you are completing the activity in someone's house, you are going to want to have it all ready to go!

- Do not focus on the outcome of the project. It does not matter that the painting didn't come out the way you expected. The real goal is to ensure that the individual enjoys the task.

- If you have a group of residents and the members of the group have varying degrees of dementia, you will want to break the task down differently for the different people. For example, if Mary is further along in her dementia than Jill, you will want to make sure that Mary's paint is already chosen for her. You thereby cut out a step that could derail her progress before she even starts if she had to do it.

- And last but not least, always ask "for help" when starting the task. Do not ask the person living with dementia if they want to paint but rather ask them if they can help you paint. People are much more likely to participate if they feel it is for a good cause, like assisting another person.

A little creativity goes a long way. There is evidence that creating art improves cognition and can improve mood in dementia. In a 2013 study, Bree Chancellor, Angel Duncan, and Anjan Chatterjee concluded that art is a positive and useful therapy in dementia care. A 2018 special edition of the journal *Dementia* (vol. 17) dedicated to exploring the role of arts in dementia suggests that creative activities not only provide an opportunity for people with dementia to express their own emotions and feelings but also facilitate communication and help foster caregivers' empathy.

EXAMPLES OF CRAFTS

Paint Birdhouses

Painting birdhouses, mini or regular sized, is an excellent craft for people with dementia (figure 19.1). The birdhouses almost always come out looking nice. People with dementia see purpose in the craft; the birdhouses get decorated and might also end up housing birds.

This craft calls for only nonwashable paint, paintbrushes, and birdhouses, so it is easy to set up and clean up. Be sure to have everything set up before inviting the person or people with dementia in to begin. Ask which colors they'd like to use and then pour the paint for them. Some people with dementia may need you to show them how to get started, but nearly everyone can continue on with this simple task once it is started.

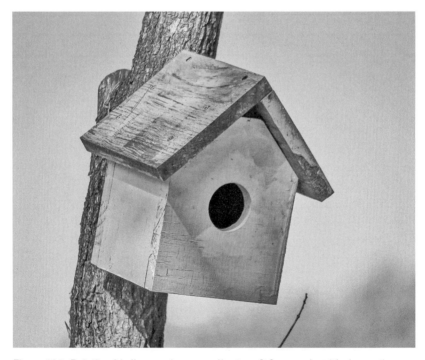

Figure 19.1. Painting birdhouses is an excellent craft for people with dementia

Tape Art

These paintings always come out looking great. Crafts that are hard to do incorrectly work well with people who have dementia. Even when someone doesn't know that they have a cognitive impairment, they may feel uncomfortable with a complicated art project. Showing a before and after picture often does the trick here.

For this craft, you'll need paint, brushes, canvas, and painter's tape (figure 19.2). Put painter's tape on the canvas in different directions. Think of it as a tie-dyeing craft—it doesn't need to have a specific pattern for it to look nice. Invite the person or people living with dementia in once everything is set up. Ask which colors they'd like to use and then pour the paint for them. Show the person with dementia how to avoid the blue painter's tape but explain that it is perfectly okay to paint on top of it by accident. Once the painting is completely dry, pull the painter's tape off.

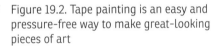

Figure 19.2. Tape painting is an easy and pressure-free way to make great-looking pieces of art

Paint a Picture of a Flower Arrangement

Telling someone living with dementia to paint a picture is too complicated and open ended of a request. Instead, many people fare better when given a specific object to paint.

For this activity, you will need flower arrangements (real or fake is fine), canvas, paint, and paintbrushes (figure 19.3). Have the flower arrangements created already or have the flowers out and ask the person to create an arrangement. Suggest that you are in need of new artwork and ask the person to help you paint a picture of the flowers in front of them.

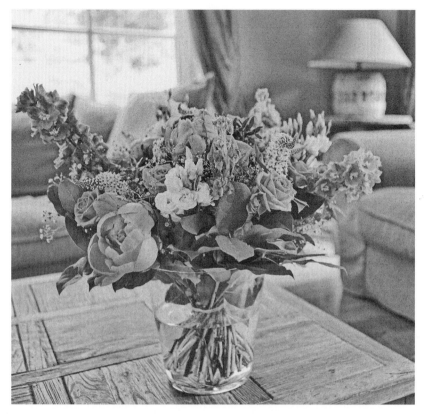

Figure 19.3. Asking a person with dementia to paint a specific object, such as a flower arrangement, helps them stay focused on the task

Draw a Memory: Your House Growing Up

Again, you want to avoid asking a person with dementia to just paint something. This is too open ended, so instead ask the person to paint a picture of the house they grew up in (figure 19.4). This engages long-term memories, helps facilitate conversation, and may even open up some interesting topics that you may not have known the person was able to talk about.

You'll need canvas, paint, and paintbrushes. Lay out the canvas and ask the person with dementia to think about the home they grew up in. Ask them to paint a picture of that house for you.

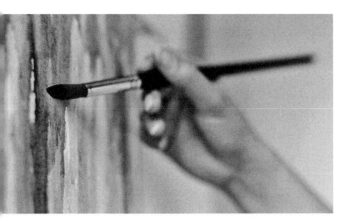

Figure 19.4. Painting childhood homes engages long-term memories and facilitates conversation

Walker Bags

It can be a real challenge to carry items when you're also pushing a walker (figure 19.5). Walker bags are functional and useful.

You'll need canvas bags, paint and/or markers, stamping materials, and string to tie the bag to the walker. Lay out the blank canvas bags, but attach one to a walker so the person can see what it will look like when finished. Ask them to design the bag however they'd like, and keep in mind that you may need to assist them a little bit. If this is in a community setting, write residents' names on the bags. Let each bag dry, and then attach it to the walker with string. Be sure that it does not get in the way of the walker wheels.

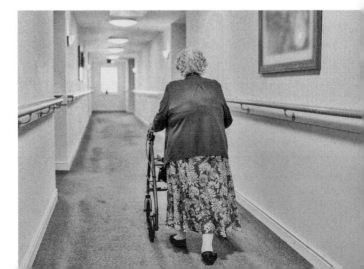

Figure 19.5. Making walker bags is a fun and useful activity for people living with dementia

SEASONAL IDEAS

Winter: A Gingerbread House

Gingerbread houses are a great winter craft! Premade gingerbread houses often work best (figure 19.6). It is also important to ensure that the person's diet will allow them to eat what they will be creating. For example, someone on a puree diet probably shouldn't do this craft: they may try to eat the candy, which could be dangerous.

Purchase premade gingerbread houses, icing, and candy, and set out butter knives for applying icing and smoothing. Ensure in advance that the icing is soft enough and easy enough to apply. If you're doing this activity in a group setting, you may want to pair residents up together. Ensure that hands are clean and washed if anyone is snacking while creating.

Figure 19.6. Premade gingerbread houses allow you to focus on decorating instead of baking and building

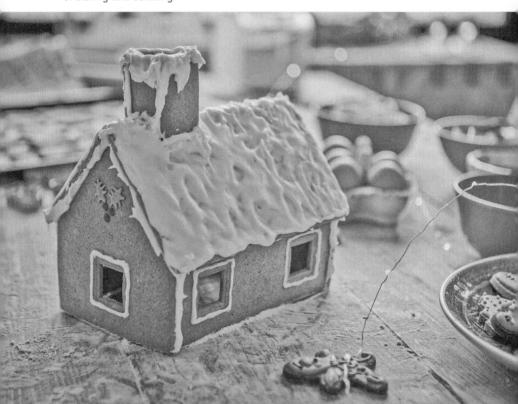

Summer: Birdfeeders

This is a great summer craft because you can complete it outside. This can be done with paper towel / toilet paper rolls or aluminum cans and fabric (as seen in figure 19.7). Filling the can with birdseed usually gets messy, so it is easier to complete in a place where you can easily toss the feed.

This activity also calls for paint, paintbrushes, string, scissors, and birdseed. Have the paint and birdseed ready to go, but prompt the person with dementia to paint and then add birdseed. This can also be a two-day activity; the painting can be on the first day and the birdseed can be added to the rolls or cans on the second. Hang the finished rolls or cans from trees that are visible from indoors (figure 19.7).

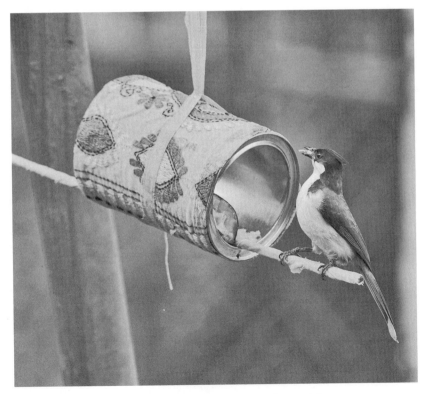

Figure 19.7. Birdfeeders can be made from a variety of materials

Spring: Flower Suncatchers

These "suncatchers" look great in a garden. It's easy to encourage creativity on this project, along with the ability to demonstrate a clear purpose in making these.

You'll need clear plastic plates, hot glue, a hot glue gun, wooden dowels, paint, and paintbrushes. You are going to be the person in charge of the hot glue gun, so set it somewhere to preheat that is safe and out of the way. Ask the person with dementia to paint the top part of the plate (the part that you would normally eat off of), including the rim if they want, and let it dry (figure 19.8). Take the wooden dowels and, using the hot glue gun, apply the dowels to the back of the plates. Stick the suncatchers in a nice spot in the garden.

Figure 19.8. Making suncatchers is a great activity that looks wonderful hanging in a garden

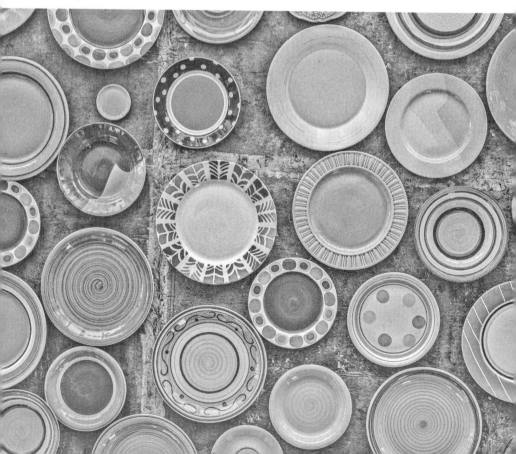

Fall: Button Trees

This is a simple craft for most people living with dementia. The objective is to add "leaves" to a tree that has been drawn onto a canvas. These leaves are three-dimensional buttons, and it gives the canvas a really unique look (figure 19.9).

This craft requires canvas, markers, glue, and buttons. Depending on the person's cognitive level, you can either draw the tree ahead of time or ask the person to draw it on the canvas. Using regular glue (not hot glue), show them how to apply a button on top of the tree drawing to look like a leaf. For people who have trouble with choosing a button, lay out a few options for them to choose from.

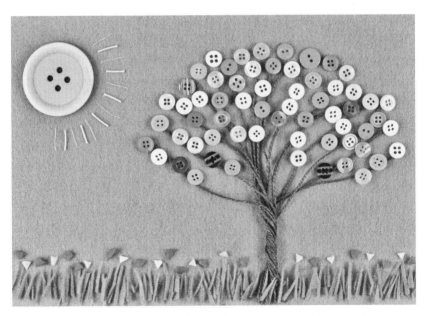

Figure 19.9. Button trees are a simple craft for most people with dementia

20

Outings

"I don't know, I think I'll just stay here," Penelope said, smiling apprehensively. "Thanks anyway." Penelope was one of our higher-functioning residents, and she loved staying busy. Crafts, games, outings, you name it—she liked to be there. Still, it was generally very difficult to get Penelope out the door for an outing, particularly if the weather wasn't perfect. When asked to join an outing, she would often become overwhelmed and misunderstand the question. Even though she always had a great time once we were out, getting her to agree to come along was a challenge. The key, we finally realized, was not to ask her if she wanted to join; instead, we started assuming that she'd come along. "Hi, Penelope, come with me," I would say. "Where are we going?" she'd ask, smiling and taking my outstretched hand. "We're going to get some ice cream at a nearby place; I know you'll have a great time," I'd reply. "Oh! Wonderful! I like ice cream," Penelope would say back.

I had asked her to join us only five minutes earlier and been declined. With a small change in phrasing, however, Penelope's attitude changed as well. She was newly excited about the possibility of an outing. Instead of giving her a chance to tell us no by asking her a question, we started with a statement.

Family members and professional care staff alike will often tell me that the person with dementia they are caring for doesn't like to go out. Occasionally, they are correct: some people do not like to go out.

And sometimes it isn't appropriate to take that individual on an outing. Generally, however, most people with dementia enjoy trips and lunch dates: they just need to be approached in the right way. In this chapter, we cover some tips and tricks to having a happy, successful outing with a person who is living with dementia.

WHEN IT MAY NOT WORK TO TRY AN OUTING

There are a few reasons why you might abstain from taking a person with dementia on an outing.

1. Their mobility issues make it a real challenge. If they are in a wheelchair and you do not have a wheelchair-accessible vehicle or a way to fold it up and put the chair in the car, an outing may be difficult. Mobility also becomes an issue if the person you want to take out has recently had a bad fall, surgery, or gets tired too quickly. Unless you are going somewhere where they can immediately sit and getting in and out of the car is not too challenging, it may not be worth taking them out.

2. Their mood is unpredictable. If the person that you wish to take on an outing has an unpredictable mood, the event could sour very quickly. Bear in mind that it is okay if the person has some bizarre social habits: that is explainable, and most passersby will understand. However, if they often flip from being overly excited to being overly irritable or anxious, bringing them to a crowded venue may be a challenge.

3. They have recently started on a new medication. If you are not sure how the new medication affects them yet, it is not wise to go too far away from home. Medication changes can deeply affect a person's mood, gait, wakefulness, frequency of need to urinate, and more.

4. The weather is poor. I have been on many an outing with people who have dementia, and I can tell you that bad weather is a big deterrent to a fun event. Most people get frustrated when it's pouring rain, and people with dementia are no different. They may be more irritable, and it is also more dangerous walking when it's slippery and damp.

5. The person is very incontinent. If the person you are looking to take out is incontinent and cannot control their bladder or bowels, a fun trip can quickly turn stressful. Particularly if you are alone and taking out more than one person living with dementia, one incontinent individual can disrupt the entire outing.

OUTINGS YOU SHOULD NOT ATTEMPT

It was one of my first times planning an excursion for my residents, and I was excited to be taking them to the North Carolina Zoo. I myself had never been to the zoo there in Asheboro, so I didn't realize how much walking was involved. In turn, I gravely underestimated how quickly my ten residents with dementia would become overwhelmed and exhausted. Even Dot, forever steady on her feet, quickly asked for a wheelchair. Lucille and Tim needed wheelchairs, too. Suddenly, nearly every one of my residents needed to be pushed in a wheelchair. Even though I had four staff members with me, I realized pretty quickly that I should have brought even more along; perhaps, even ten, so that I would have had a one-to-one ratio. Needless to say, we didn't stay at the zoo very long.

There are some outings you should not attempt. The person you are planning to take out will determine which sorts of outings you should or should not attempt. Here is a short list of some of the outings you may want to reconsider.

1. Any trip that may involve too much walking. It's best to find a location that has a small loop that you can take, so that the group does not end up too far from the entry and exit points.

2. Going to their old house. Taking a person to see the house they used to live in is unkind and irresponsible unless the person completely understands that it is not their house anymore and that they live elsewhere. I have seen many caregivers use a trip to an old house as a way to "convince" a person with dementia that they can no longer live there. This should never be the reason that they visit their old stomping grounds. For many people living with dementia, seeing an old house confuses them and causes pain rather than brings relief and makes them happy.

3. Going to the cemetery to visit deceased loved ones. Again, unless the person with dementia knows that their loved ones have passed and they've specifically asked to visit the grave site, this type of trip is unwise. Many people with dementia, especially those in moderate or later stages of the disease, become confused about who is still alive and who has passed away. Taking someone to the cemetery to show them that a certain loved one is dead often causes anxiety and pain.

4. Funeral. It is not a good idea to take people with dementia to funerals for the same reason it is not generally a good idea to take a person with dementia to a cemetery. Unless they live with both their feet in our reality, and they believe and understand that a person has passed away, a funeral is often an overwhelming and confusing event for a person with dementia.

5. A huge event like a wedding. While weddings can be fun, they can also be very overwhelming. Consider the individual's stage of dementia before embarking on a big event like this: if they are in a later stage of dementia, they may become tired and restless very quickly. Added noise, partygoers, and excitement could combine to make this kind of outing very challenging. The same thing goes for holiday parties. I think it is a great idea to bring a loved one with dementia to your place for family holiday gatherings, but it may be wise to create a plan that will let you isolate them from the noise and partygoers if they get overwhelmed.

6. Places that do not have a nearby restroom. Particularly if more than one person with dementia is accompanying you on your outing, the bathroom situation can quickly become a real issue. The last thing you want to be doing is waiting in line for a toilet if the person you are with desperately needs to use it.

7. Isolated places where if the person fell or needed assistance, you might not be able to help them by yourself. A trip to the local creek where they used to fish could be wonderful—or it could quickly take a turn for the worse. Bring someone else with you if you are taking a person living with dementia to a more isolated spot.

TIPS FOR A GREAT OUTING

Will had been a teacher his whole adult life. He absolutely loved working with kids, particularly children younger than 10. That's why when we started planning our trip to the local preschool, we knew Will would be on board. We gathered up a group of residents who would enjoy the trip and hopped on the bus to the preschool.

The teachers at the preschool were thrilled to see us. Our residents would be reading to their students, as they did twice a month. The kids looked forward to it too. The beautiful thing about this outing was that these 2- and 3-year-olds did not realize our residents had cognitive deficits, as many older children would have. We let our residents take turns reading to the kids, but I had a secret fear that Will would want to read. I didn't want him to become embarrassed, as I believed that he could no longer read.

One day, my growing concern became a reality. "Can I read to the kids?" he asked. I felt my stomach drop, but I nodded. "Of course!" I said, smiling, and handed him the book. Will sat back down and faced the kids. "Okay, kids!" he started. "Today we're going to be reading about Sally and her trip to the store. How many of you go with your parents to the store?" Will surveyed the class. The kids started raising their hands, calling out, "Me! Me!" I noticed a teacher in the back gently wipe her eyes with the back of her hand.

"Sally wanted to go to the store and buy three apples," Will read. "Now, kids, how many apples did she want to buy?" he asked, quizzing them about what they'd just heard. "Three!" the preschoolers crooned back. Chills shot through me: this was the most wonderful thing I had ever seen. Clearly, I had underestimated Will's skillset.

While there are a few places that you should not attempt to take people with dementia, there are far more that are excellent choices. Restaurant trips, ice cream outings, a fun car or bus ride, a trip to the store, a trip to a kindergarten or preschool classroom, or a visit to an animal shelter are all great ideas. Here are a few tips that can help to make an outing successful.

1. Always plan ahead of time. Visit the location that you are planning to take the person or persons with dementia to, preferably during the time you had planned to take the trip. Is there ample

parking? Will the location become too crowded? Are there better times of day for you to take them there? Is there an easy way to exit the location in case of an emergency? These are all excellent questions to consider when choosing an excursion.

2. Pack extra items that you may need. Snacks, water, extra adult briefs, and even the person's medication are items you will want to bring along.

3. If you are going to a restaurant for lunch, let the person or persons with dementia look at the menu. After a couple minutes, take the menu away and offer two or three choices. A large menu can be very overwhelming for someone who has trouble making choices. While it's great to let the person keep a sense of normalcy by reviewing the menu, it is best to then take the list and narrow it down for them.

4. Bring along some personalized business cards that read to the effect of "Please excuse my companion. They have dementia and may need some extra assistance and patience." It may be useful to hand to people in the vicinity who seem alarmed by something the person with dementia is doing or saying.

5. Stick to a one-to-one ratio for bigger outings. If you are taking a group of residents on a bus trip and not leaving the bus, two staff members should be fine. But if you are taking a group of people on an outing, a larger number of staff members is necessary. Some residents' family members may want to come along and help: this can be a great idea and very helpful as long as they're familiar with the community's rules and regulations.

6. Consider the time of day and the length of the outing. Many people living with dementia become more restless and agitated later in the day—a syndrome called "sundowning"—so taking a trip and returning home before 1:00 pm is advised. A long

outing may also not be preferable, as it increases the likelihood that people with dementia will become exhausted and overwhelmed. One of my favorite outings for people who have dementia is an hour-long trip to get ice cream. Get in, eat ice cream, and leave, all within an hour. The number of smiling faces seems to drop if the event goes on too long.

AT HOME

If you are taking only one person with dementia on an outing, things tend to be a little easier. There are significantly fewer items you need to worry about, and there is only one person you have to attend to. Still, it is wise to know that individual well before starting on an excursion. For example, a trip to the animal shelter will not go well if Christina is allergic to cats or is afraid of dogs. If this person is your family member, you probably already know a lot about their preferences and can take these into account. If this person is in your care and is unrelated to you, it is advisable to spend a week or more with them before attempting an outing. The best thing that you can do is plan for a short, easy excursion at first. Try a trip to get ice cream and then extend it to a lunch outing. If the lunch outing goes well, try a trip to the grocery store. If that goes well, too, start looking at longer outings they may enjoy.

Consider, too, the transportation that you need. Always, always take their walker or wheelchair, even if you do not plan on leaving the car. A scenic car ride can quickly become disastrous if someone needs to use the restroom or grab a bite to eat and there is no mobility aid. The same thing goes for medication: even if you plan on returning well before it is time for them to take their medication, bring it along. Things happen, and we want to be sure that we've allowed room for human error.

IN A COMMUNITY SETTING

In a community setting, it is inevitable that you will be traveling with more than one companion. I recommend taking no fewer than six to make the trip worth it. If you are taking a bus ride and do not plan on leaving the bus, you are free to pack the seats with residents. Still, bring along at least one other staff member. We always want to be prepared for the worst: if the bus breaks down, the last thing you will want is to be the only person helping ten people living with dementia. You will also need to bring along everyone's walkers or wheelchairs. An unexpected bathroom stop can become a real challenge without everyone's walking aids.

When gathering a group for an outing, carefully consider who will be joining you. For example, if you know that Katherine and Greg don't get along, perhaps you may want to consider bringing one but not the other. If Trish and Megan don't travel without one another, you will have to bring both of them. And if Megan doesn't walk well, you may want to reconsider bringing Trish on that mall trip.

Ensure, too, that you have alerted your accompanying staff members well ahead of time. When you work in assisted living, it always seems like emergencies are popping up everywhere. The last thing you want is to be loading the bus up with residents and have your two accompanying staff members bail out at the last moment due to an unexpected move-in. Have a couple of backup staff members who can join you on the excursion.

You will also want to make three written lists of the residents who are joining you. One is for your records and to take with you and the other two are for the community. One should sit near the sign-out list, so that incoming family members can see if their loved one is out of the community. The third list should stay with the nurse or director at the community. Also, be sure to review the list with the nurse ahead of time. If someone has recently changed medications or if they need wound care, taking them on an outing would not be wise. Don't be afraid to get input from other staff members, particularly if you are unsure about which residents to take. Lastly, follow the policies that your facility has in place for removing residents. This is for their safety as well as yours.

When it's time to start getting everyone together for the trip, be sure to phrase the come-along request appropriately with your residents. With many residents, it will work best to say "Come with me" or "Help me get everyone into the front room." Some people with dementia will say no even if they'd have a great time on the trip. In order to avoid getting a lot of refusals, know how to phrase the request.

Position a staff member in the room where you will be gathering all your residents. It is always frustrating to gather a few people, leave to get more residents, and then return to a now-empty room. Many people with dementia will get up and leave when they are not sure of what is going on or where they will be going. Positioning a staff member in the room that you'll be leaving from is always the safest bet. They can ensure that your residents are entertained and not heading off back to their respective rooms.

CONCLUSION

There are about a million ways to create a successful outing, and I've listed a few that can help get you started. Most people learn as they go along, but hopefully, a few of these suggestions will help prevent you from making some of the same mistakes I have made. Outings are so important in dementia care and should not be put on the back burner. Often, you will hear that "there's not enough time" or "they don't like outings" as an excuse to avoid going outside. It's not possible to live a full life if you are stuck in the house or in the assisted living community. There are plenty of ways to help people with dementia enjoy fresh air— you may just need to be a little creative.

21

Entertainment and Home Visitors

WHAT COUNTS AS ENTERTAINMENT?

"What does this mean, 'Yoga with Katy'?" I asked my boss. It was my first job in dementia care, and I was in charge of all activities in the community. I was 24 years old, excited, and ready to work, but completely overwhelmed. "Oh, I don't know, let me see," she said, taking the calendar from me. "Hmm, right, that was our previous memory care activity manager's friend who came in to do yoga with the residents," she said, nodding and handing the calendar back to me. "Does she . . . always come in? How do we reach her?" I asked. My boss shrugged, not very invested in helping me solve this mystery. "I think there's a rolodex of names and numbers somewhere in your office; maybe the yoga friend is in there," she offered.

It would be three months before I had my activity calendars just the way I wanted them. I was fortunate to have a great, caring staff who supported most things that I put on the calendar. Truly, the most challenging task I had was hunting down and organizing the previous manager's entertainment for the community: she'd booked a number of unreliable volunteers, musical acts she hadn't paid, and people whose numbers I couldn't locate. Using a combination of the web, word of mouth, and mailings that were delivered to the community, I was able to string together a few regular acts that would come in to perform for my residents. Among my residents' favorites were a piano player, pet therapy, a local artist, a singer, an accordion player, and a dance and exercise group.

Booking entertainment for your care community can be a real challenge, but when it works out, it truly pays off. There is nothing like watching your residents with dementia get up, dance, sing, and engage in new ways, if only for a brief period of time. What counts as entertainment? Entertainment is anyone or anything that comes into the community ready to perform for your residents or lead a group in an activity that is different from what the community normally offers.

I have had local pet owners bring their therapy-certified dogs, rabbits, cats, and even iguanas into the community to visit my residents. I've been to communities where the residents' favorite entertainment was a keyboard player, and then I've been to other places where the residents absolutely adored the eclectic oldies-playing band that came in once a month. A lot depends on where your community is located, the residents' general taste in music and dance, and your residents' acuity. For example, if your residents are lower functioning, someone coming in to lead an art class may not get a positive response. If your residents love country music, but you bring in a local classic rock band, you may also not receive the desired response.

FINDING ENTERTAINMENT

I have been to a number of dementia care communities where the activity directors have said things like "We don't have a budget for entertainment" or "I can't find anyone to come see my residents," which, to me, seem like excuses. With a little bit of hard work and some elbow grease, any community can create at least a small outside entertainment list for their residents. If money is the problem, petition the community's decision makers for an entertainment budget. If that doesn't work, find volunteers, such as local college or high school students looking to put in some volunteer hours. One of the best ways to find entertainment is to ask residents' family members. I can say this works for certain, because I've always been a transplant: coming from another state or part of the state and starting work at a new community, I have never known who or where to call in order to locate entertainment, but with a little asking around, I have always found reliable performers and group leaders.

Don't be afraid to ask reliable friends for assistance too. Maybe you have a friend who plays guitar really well, and she'd be interested in volunteering once or twice a month for an hour. New, happy faces are always great invites to your senior living community. Children especially work wonders when it comes to bringing up spirits. Local elementary schools often do small plays or talent shows during the holidays. See if a local school would be interested in coming by to sing for your residents. Even honor society groups at local high schools are great places to look for volunteers. One of the most valuable things I have ever done, to this day, was a small project I undertook my senior year of high school. A week after prom, I gathered a group of fifteen or twenty students together and traveled to a local skilled nursing facility in our prom dresses and suits. We did a "fashion show" for their residents, and I will never forget the tears of joy the residents shed.

The point is this: it should not be that difficult to find entertainment. Sometimes, especially without a budget, you may just need to get a tad creative.

SCHEDULING ENTERTAINMENT

"But Dance Beats Dance Troupe has always come here at 6:30!" one of my staff members said. "The residents like it that way," she added, nodding and pointing to the five residents waiting for the performance to start. Truly, it didn't make any sense the way that it was set up. In fact, I had a feeling that the previous activity director had set it up this way so that she could leave work early. No matter the reason, I had to change the time. By 6:30 pm, most of my residents had finished dinner and retired to their rooms. Most of them woke up around 5 am, so 6:30 pm without a nap was quite a full day. Although a few of them enjoyed the later entertainment, for many, the noise was far too loud. "I can't hear my TV!" Mattie yelled from her room.

Scheduling entertainment involves two tasks: finding out when your performer is available and then comparing that with the times of day that are best for your residents. For example, you would not want to schedule a musician for 6 pm, as most of your residents are going to be tired and potentially agitated by this point in the day. Bringing in an influx of noise and people to the common living area is going to elicit a lot of undesirable reactions.

Performers may offer to perform for an extended period of time, but you should typically decline this offer. Most people living with dementia become bored or agitated with any performance that lasts longer than an hour.

It's also important to do a trial run with the performer before committing to bringing them in for the long term. See how your residents like them and see how the performer does with your residents, and if it seems to be working, then figure out if the time of day is feasible going forward. It's best to get the entertainer on a regular monthly schedule. It was always nice to know that our piano player would be there every first and third Tuesday of the month.

GETTING EVERYONE READY FOR THE SHOW

Once the event is on your calendar, ensure that the staff knows about it. Your management team and care staff team should be aware of big events before they happen; it's especially important to remind them on the day of the event that it is happening. They can help you bring residents to the event, and they can ensure that families know about it as well. Families can see just how positive dementia care communities can be on those days when musicians or dance groups come in to perform.

Gathering a big group of residents can sometimes be a challenge. Ask for other staff members' assistance in bringing residents into the common area where the performance will be happening. Try not to bring anyone into the space before the performer arrives: you will no doubt lose almost everyone after only a few minutes when they realize nothing is happening. As the entertainment is setting up, start bringing in your residents who are least likely to leave or become frustrated. The residents who are the most easily distracted should join the group last, once entertainment has already begun.

COPING WITH DIFFICULT PERFORMERS

"The residents keep taking my bongos," Shannon said, standing at my office door. "Um . . . don't you give your bongos to them so that they can play along with your music?" I asked slowly, turning to face her. "Yeah, I do, but then I need them back, and some of your patients have left the room with them!" she explained, clearly frustrated.

This wasn't the first time that Shannon had complained to me about something that was really quite normal in dementia care. "Here's the thing," I said. "All of my residents have dementia, and this is going to happen. If you give them something, they may walk off with it. It's okay. It's normal. It's okay that this annoys you, but if you continue to have issues like this, I think you might want to consider giving up this gig. Maybe this isn't a good fit."

She paused, surprised that I'd say this. "Oh, well, I guess . . . I guess it's okay that they take the bongos for a little bit. I'll get them back," she said, now focused on the fact that she didn't want to lose a paying client.

I did eventually fire this entertainer: she was a lot more drama than she was worth.

Not everyone is good at dementia care. While the large majority of performers that I've hired in my career are excellent, kind, and patient with my residents, not everyone is. Working with people who are living with dementia requires a certain level of patience and understanding that not everyone possesses, and that is okay. Don't be afraid to remove someone from your performer list if they seem as though they don't understand how to communicate with your residents. First, try educating them. Offer some constructive criticism and teach them about dementia and brain changes that they may notice. If this doesn't work, a dementia care community probably is not a good fit for them. It is far better to fire someone who doesn't understand dementia and your residents than to keep them on for the sake of having another performer.

AT HOME

What Counts as a New Visitor or Entertainment?

Chantel arrived, guitar under her arm. She was from a local volunteer organization that catered to seniors and had seen Ellen's name and information online. "Hi, Ellen!" Chantel greeted her as she walked through the door. "I'm with In Service of Seniors. I heard you love music," she said, smiling. Ellen was surprised: she hadn't remembered that any visitors were coming today, but this young woman seemed kind. "Yes, I like music," Ellen replied, offering Chantel a seat. Chantel stayed for an hour, playing some of Ellen's favorite old songs and singing along with her.

Normally when we think of entertainment, we think of it as someone coming in to perform for residents in a care community setting, but it can also mean visitors to the home. These could be volunteers who come to play music for the person at home, or they could even be out-of-town family members stopping by for the afternoon. Home care is a great option for a lot of people with dementia, but it can definitely become isolating after a while. Even if a home care agency is sending in new faces every couple of days, it's still one-on-one care. A new face in the way of entertainment or simply a visit can be a welcome change. Meals on Wheels of America is a fantastic organization that brings by meals for at-home seniors. While they are there to bring a meal, they are also checking in on the individual to make sure that they seem healthy and safe. It can be a welcome sight for a person with dementia who sees the same faces every day.

SCHEDULING VISITORS

It is worth noting that visitors and entertainers cannot take the place of the caregiver. I have occasionally met family members who bring in a volunteer to sit with their loved one with dementia in the hope that that will permit them to get out for the afternoon. But unless someone is trained (and licensed) in the care of a person with dementia, it's not safe to leave them alone with a person who cannot care for themselves.

The time at which you schedule visitors, be they family members of the person with dementia, entertainers, volunteers, or even hospice nurses, will depend a lot on the individual with dementia's waking hours. If they are most awake and lively in the early afternoon, schedule visitors for this time of day. You would not want people coming in and trying to communicate or get information from the person living with dementia when they are exhausted or overwhelmed. If the person with dementia is protective of their house and possessions, visitors may not be welcome at all. For example, if a home care agency has a hard enough time getting themselves in the door, sending more people to "visit" may be a bad idea.

COPING WITH DIFFICULT VISITORS

"Aunt Lisa!" Harold called down the hall. "Remember me? I'm your nephew, Harold!" Oh, fantastic, Lisa's home caregiver thought. Every time he visits, he upsets his aunt. "Yes, hi, Harold," Lisa replied, taking his hand. "Last time, you couldn't remember my name, re-member that?" he asked his aunt. "Seems like your dementia has gotten better!"

Most people who approach people with dementia this way generally just need a little bit of dementia education. If you are from a home care agency and the person causing a disturbance is a relative of the person with dementia, talk to your supervisor at work. See if there's a way that they can address the issue with the family in a professional way. If you are a loved one of the person with dementia, don't be afraid to lay down the law of the land. There is a way to be polite but also firm when speaking to individuals who don't understand dementia care. Sometimes a good example will do the trick. Saying something like "If you were confused about who your visitors were, would you want someone to make you feel bad by pointing that out?" It can be difficult for people with no dementia care background to understand what people with dementia feel and need.

Sensory Rooms and Activity Boxes

WHAT IS A SENSORY ROOM?

Makoto was easily overwhelmed by large groups of people, especially since he had progressed further into dementia. Because he was not very mobile on his own, Makoto spent much of his time in a comfortable recliner chair. Generally, he was very pleasant and played games and did activities with the rest of the group. Especially in the evening, however, as he began to sundown, Makoto would start to cry out for his wife. He often hallucinated and would sometimes see her among the other residents.

The staff was unsure of what to do: they could not bring him back to his room, for fear that he might try to get up and end up falling. They also found that bringing him outside and away from the noise didn't help much: he was then overwhelmed by all the sights, noises, and lights outdoors. After I studied the room a bit, I suggested turning Makoto's chair just slightly to face the window. He could still be in the room with other residents, but his general gaze would face the garden that he loved.

As it turned out, this slight shift in the positioning of Makoto's chair helped immensely. Once the big group of residents in his line of vision was no longer in his line of vision, he became much calmer and happier.

In my work as a consultant, I've gotten many requests for sensory rooms and for sensory and activity boxes. A sensory room is a space that is built to be a controlled sensory environment. Like Makoto, many people with dementia can become overwhelmed when there is too much going on around them. The sensory room offers a separate space that features calming lights, sounds, and objects. This same type of therapy is often offered for people—and especially children—with autism. Sometimes these spaces have sound machines or provide soft, calming things to touch, like sand or faux fur.

Any space can become a sensory room. You don't necessarily need a bubble machine or a waterfall sounds CD to make the room work. In Makoto's case, we didn't even need a sensory room: we just had to adjust his position slightly. This is to suggest that you can create a calm, welcoming environment inside your house or in a care community setting without changing much at all. Truly, the goal is to offer a space where someone with dementia can go to get away from what is happening nearby them. I recommend having this option available even at family gatherings, where hours-long parties and big crowds can create challenging situations for people with dementia. An extra, quiet bedroom down the hall can provide this type of environment.

HOW DO YOU INTRODUCE A SENSORY ROOM?

Note that when I say "sensory room," I am also referring to calming, quiet spaces. These can be a space in the same room the person with dementia normally spends time in or another room that is not being used.

Ideally, you want to bring a person living with dementia to a sensory room *before* they become agitated and stressed. Sometimes it can be hard to tell if someone is going to get upset, but if you look for certain triggers, it isn't usually too difficult to predict. For example, if Renee gets upset only in the later afternoon, you know that it may be better to bring her to the sensory room before and right after dinner. This sets

Renee up for success: she's calmed down before dinner starts, and after dinner, when she starts feeling anxious again, she is back in the sensory room, starting an activity by herself.

Do not ask the person with dementia if they want to go with you to the sensory room; just say something like "Follow me" or "Let's go over here," even if they are in a wheelchair and need to be brought to the room. Make sure you always introduce the action before you start it, even if the person cannot actually initiate action without your assistance.

It's a lot easier to simply prevent or minimize anxiety than to stop it once a person has begun to experience it. It does happen sometimes, though, that you will have to battle the agitation when it's in full swing. Recognize that a sensory room is not always going to solve the problem. Recognize too that even though the room worked last week, it will not necessarily work this week. Dementia care is trial and error as much as it is practice and knowing the individual: you may have to try a few things before you find something that works. If Renee is already agitated, tell her to come with you, and then head to the sensory room. Begin an activity with her or perhaps just sit calmly. If she is inconsolable, and it's because she's overwhelmed, sit behind her so she cannot see you. She may be more agitated with you in her line of vision.

Do not leave the person with dementia in the room by themselves with the door closed. If someone is agitated—or even if they aren't—they could be a fall or injury risk if left alone. If no one is available to remain in the room with the person, then even if they are screaming or crying, keep the door open. Closing the door to "keep everyone else calm" or "calm them down" is not a safe practice. You want to ensure that someone has eyes on that person or that at least people are regularly walking by the room to make sure they are safe.

Beyond all else, stay calm. The worst thing that you can do is panic because that is likely to make the person with dementia panic even more. Take a few deep breaths and know that their agitation will pass; it may just take a bit of time.

A recent review of the research (Lorusso & Bosch, 2018) on the use of multisensory rooms found that the quality of life for patients with dementia was positively impacted by most who used them, but we do not yet know how long the effects last or how long or often someone needs to use them to experience a positive result. There's also no current research indicating that the use of these rooms is always better than reading to someone with dementia or simply talking with them, that is, engaging in one-on-one interactions. But what is important is that using these rooms is another nonpharmacological tool available for you to use to help persons with dementia, especially given that it can be challenging to provide enough one-on-one engagement in care facilities. Keep in mind that they are rather simple and inexpensive to create and that they may work for some people with dementia, although not necessarily on every occasion.

WHAT ARE ACTIVITY BOXES?

While we believed that at least half of Makoto's outbursts and panic later in the day were due to overstimulation, we also had a hunch that the other half were due to his boredom. Some activities were too challenging for Makoto to participate in, so he would sit in his chair near the window. When Makoto's family used to care for him at home, they'd often find him reading the newspaper or organizing mail. "Dad likes to be busy," his daughter told the staff. In order to keep him engaged, they began to create boxes of premade activities. Because their father really enjoyed reading through and sorting letters and newspapers, the family put together a box full of old letters, cards, and newspaper clippings. It was not clear exactly what Makoto was doing when he was sorting, but it was quite evident that he was happy organizing everything. If disturbed during his mission, he would look up, a confused smile on his face, surprised that he'd been interrupted. Knowing that Makoto liked to be busy, we began putting together activity boxes to use with him and the other residents.

Activity boxes, engagement boxes, life skill boxes—or whatever you'd like to call them—are an integral part of successful dementia care setup for both in-home care and care communities. If you are offering dementia care, you need activity boxes. The point of these boxes is to provide a premade, easy-to-use activity for individuals who have dementia. Care staff or family members should be able to pull out the box, open it up, and immediately start on the activity with minimal instructions. Unlike a craft, game, or physical exercise, these activities are built to require little to no setup or supervision. You should be able to set up the activity box with the individual who has dementia and then go about your other tasks (Guwaldi, 2013).

One important note: if you are planning to create a sensory or reminiscing box, be sure that the person who has dementia is not inclined to put inedible items in their mouth. Most people living with dementia will not do this. However, someone who is very advanced may confuse a box of buttons (great for plunging hands into and feeling around) with something edible. Be sure that this is not an issue before walking away from the individual.

If you are creating a reminiscing box, such as a box full of sand and seashells, you may want to sit beside the person with whom you are sharing it. Reminiscing boxes can provide great opportunities for conversation. If you are making this for staff members, type up a list of questions and put this in the box. Conversation starters like "What is your favorite thing about the beach?" or "Did you ever play any water sports?" are great options for this type of activity. Feeling sand between their fingers and touching seashells may open up a world of conversation you hadn't previously thought possible.

The easiest way to put these boxes together is head to a dollar store or other large retailer. You will want to find bins that come with lids, and ones that fit easily into a closet or bookshelf. Then, you can go about getting creative with what to put in each box. Some of my favorite examples of activity box items include the following:

- Socks to match and sort

- Hand towels to fold

- Silverware to organize

- Poker chips to stack

- Baby clothes to fold

- Holiday cards to sort

- Faux flowers to arrange into vases

- Clothespins to clip on a clothesline

- Plastic Easter eggs to put together

- Sensory and reminiscing box options: sand, seashells, dried flowers, buttons, photos, etc.

There are a ton of examples of great activity boxes, and I am sure that you can think of many that are not on this list. The activities in each box are easy to explain to someone with dementia: they require almost no instruction. Most of these things, like folding, sorting, and matching, come naturally to us—we've been doing them our whole lives, and they're firmly planted in our long-term memories. People living with dementia do not quickly lose their ability to do these simple tasks, but you may need to modify the task slightly. For some individuals, giving them one hand towel at a time is perfect. For others, you can dump the whole basket on the table and they are able to fold all of them without difficulty. The best thing about these activity boxes is that they are so simple to use. Staff or families are able to pull out the box, ask the person with dementia "for help" with the activity, and then move on about their day. While most of these items will only keep people with dementia engaged for a maximum of thirty minutes, that's thirty minutes that they are active and interested in something other than watching television or napping.

HOW DO YOU INTRODUCE AN ACTIVITY BOX?

One of the main points I make in this book is that if you ask someone with a cognitive impairment if they want to do something, you are approaching them the wrong way. Instead, you need to ask that person "for help" or if they can "come with you" to do something. Many of the activity boxes have the person with dementia performing tasks that recall daily chores around the house. These chores work well because everyone is familiar with them, and because once the chores are completed, most people feel good about themselves. We want to ensure that we set people with dementia up for success! A fantastic way to do that is to provide them with things that we know they can do with very little outside help.

There are a number of ways to get the person interested in the activity boxes. You can start by asking, "Can you help me?" and then show them what you need help with. If your person with dementia is occupied doing something else, like watching TV, extend a hand and say, "I really need your help. Can you come help me?" Most protests like "Oh, I don't think so" or "I don't know" come from a place of insecurity. The person may be very aware of the fact that they haven't been able to accomplish tasks in the past and may be concerned that they will fail again. You can say things like "I heard you're really quick and good at folding towels" or "I'm so busy; I think you're the only person who can help me finish this" to get them involved. The goal is to make that person feel as important and necessary as possible by getting them invested in the task. Most people are very unlikely to turn down a chance to help another, especially if they are made feel they are the most appropriate person to assist.

Silvester sat watching TV, although his head nodded slightly up and down as though he was beginning to drift off to sleep. I walked over and approached the couch, sitting down low beside it. "Hey, Silvester," I said, smiling and gently touching his arm to ensure he was aware of me. He looked up and matched my smile. "Hi," he said, sleepily. "Can you help me with something?" I asked him. "Oh . . . I don't think I will be good at that," Silvester replied, shaking his head, even though he wasn't sure what the task was yet. "You know," I started. "I heard that you're really great at organizing silverware, and that's good news for me, because I have a ton of silverware I need to sort. I could really use your help!" I watched as Silvester considered this. "Okay, I can try," he said.

I walked Silvester over to the nearest table where I'd already laid out the silverware. "I have a lot to do today and it's going to be so helpful to have you finish this for me!" I smiled. He smiled back and sat down to work on it. Immediately, he was organizing silverware into piles. Most people don't find this type of task to be engaging or fun, but for someone with dementia, being asked to participate can mean a lot. I made sure that Silvester felt confident about his task and then quietly walked away. I checked back in a few minutes to find him hard at work and with a small smile on his face.

You can introduce an activity box at any time, but I find that they are best used throughout the day to "fill in the gaps" when there's nothing else going on. Say you have lunch planned, an outing, and then some downtime. Keeping the person with dementia busy is imperative: it prevents them from sleeping too much, getting bored, or becoming

irritable. I have also used them when I have had a large group of residents with dementia with different levels of functioning. In that sce-
nario, I will take my higher-functioning residents and start them on a
task and then provide my other residents with the boxes. Whether for
use in downtime or for helping with keeping certain members of diverse
groups engaged, I make activity boxes part of the daily plan.

IN A COMMUNITY SETTING

Sensory Rooms

Sensory rooms, or multisensory environments, have been used with
people with dementia since the early 1990s. Dementia impacts the ability of those affected to regulate their own sensory stimulation, and so
they can become easily over- or understimulated (Lorusso & Bosch,
2018). There have been many anecdotal reports about their effectiveness, but research has been somewhat scarce, and some care providers
in fact fear that research could have a negative impact on the "human-
istic and patient-centered philosophy" that underlies their use (Hope,
1998, p. 378). Kevin Hope, a gerontologist and nurse, examines ways in
which they are most effective in a 1998 study. The study notes that most
patients with dementia were calmed and soothed by the experience and
became more likely to want to interact with, and be more cooperative
with, others. But multisensory environments didn't work for everyone.
Hope also emphasizes that staff in care facilities should be trained in
how to use these spaces and not treat them as simply time-out rooms
when people with dementia become anxious. He even suggests that
multisensory rooms be used on a regular, planned, and therapeutic
basis rather than on an as-needed basis. The systematic review of the
literature by Lesa Lorusso and Sheila Bosch (2018) also finds that quality of life for patients with dementia is positively impacted by most who
use the multisensory rooms, but we do not yet know how long lasting
the effects are or if they work better than other types of treatment.

I built a space like this in an assisted living building in Pittsburgh. They had a very small room to work with and wanted it to be a sensory space. I purchased the following items for them: a bookshelf and baskets to hold simple puzzles and games, a bubble machine for the wall, a garden scene painting that played pond sounds behind it, faux grass to touch and feel, a large wall sticker of a tree and three-dimensional birdhouses to affix to the wall, and a table and chairs. The community had a lot of residents who were advanced in their dementia, so the room offered a quiet space where residents could sit with one or two other individuals to relax.

Activity Boxes

In a community setting, I train my staff on how to best utilize the activity boxes. Often, at first, there is some dismay regarding the use of the boxes. "I don't have time" or "I don't think the residents will like these" are some of the first things you might hear from staff members. The best part about these boxes for staff, though, is that they give them *more* time: residents are less bored and more engaged, so there tends to be less falling and less-frequent bathroom requests. Five minutes is all it takes to set up an activity box and get residents engaged.

Putting this type of activity on the calendar is a snap. Because of many residents' memory impairments, you can also use these boxes more than once a day. They are great pre- or postmeal activities because they take so little time to set up. Residents can even sit at their mealtime seats and fold towels, sort socks, or arrange flowers.

In a group or with an individual resident, the key, as always, is to ask them "for help" when starting the activity. Approaching a table and asking them if they want to match socks is probably going to get a strong no from the group.

AT HOME

Even at home, activity boxes are useful to keep around. I have sometimes noticed that families expect *more* engagement for the person living with dementia when there is one-on-one care. On that note, I have also observed that many home care agencies don't train their staff members in this type of engagement. "I just don't know what to do with her during the day," so many care staff members, relatives, and friends of people with dementia have said to me. Activity boxes provide a premade, easy-to-use way to engage.

These boxes are perfect for downtime, pre- or postmeals, and waking up or even while watching TV. There is no wrong way to use these activity kits, as long as you use them. Of course, ask the person "for help" when starting the activity. If you ask someone if they want to fold towels you will probably be told no. In good news, even if you get a negative answer when you ask for help, you can always try again later: their answer may be completely different.

Acknowledgments

I would like to acknowledge the contribution of Dr. Geri M. Lotze to this work. Geri reviewed all of the manuscript in draft and in final forms, made excellent suggestions regarding content changes and updates, wrote the chapter on music-based activities, ensured that all recommendations were based on sound science, and encouraged me throughout the process of writing this book. Geri was my professor for a psychology of aging class I took during college and someone who inspired me to pursue a career in the field of gerontology.

In addition, I want to acknowledge my professors in the Psychology Department at the University of Mary Washington and the Social Sciences and Gerontology departments at the University of North Carolina at Greensboro, who provided me with a strong foundation in human behavior and aging care. I am also grateful to my grandparents who showed me that aging can be graceful, happy, and full of love and wisdom.

Bibliography

Chapter 1: What Is Dementia?

Budson, A. E., & Kowall, N. W. (2014). *The handbook of Alzheimer's disease and other dementias.* West Sussex, UK: John Wiley and Sons.

Mace, N. L., & Rabins, P. V. (2017). *The 36-hour day: A family guide to caring for people who have Alzheimer disease, other dementias, and memory loss* (6th ed.). Baltimore, MD: Johns Hopkins University Press.

Chapter 2: Building a Dementia-Friendly Environment

Lawton M. P. (1983). Environment and other determinants of well-being in older people. *Gerontologist, 23:* 349–357.

Chapter 3: Caregiver Stress

American Medical Association. *Caregiver Self-Assessment Questionnaire.* https://www.caregiverslibrary.org/Portals/0/CaringforYourself _CaregiverSelfAssessmentQuestionaire.pdf.

Kiecolt-Glaser, J. K., Glaser R,. Gravenstein, S., Malarkey, W. B., Sheridan J. (1996). Chronic stress alters the immune response to influenza virus vaccine in older adults. *Proceedings of the National Academy of Sciences, 93* (7): 3043–3047.

Losada, A., Márquez-González, M., Puente, C., & Romero-Moreno, R. (2010). Development and validation of the caregiver guilt questionnaire. *International Psychogeriatrics, 22* (4): 650–660.

Roach, L., Laidlaw, K., Gillanders, D., & Quinn, K. (2013). Validation of the caregiver guilt questionnaire (CGQ) in a sample of British dementia caregivers. *International Psychogeriatrics, 25* (12): 2001–2010.

Chapter 4: Creating a Calendar

Khachiyants, N., Trinkle, D., Son, S. J., & Kim, K. Y. (2011). Sundown syndrome in persons with dementia: An update. *Psychiatry Investigation, 8* (4): 275–287.

Chapter 5: Embracing the Reality of People Living with Dementia

Blum, N. (1994). Deceptive practices in managing a family member with Alzheimer's disease. *Symbolic Interactionism, 17:* 21–36.

Cantone, D., Attena, F., Cerrone, S., Fabozzi, A., Rossiello, R., Spagnoli, L., & Pelullo, C. (2018). Lying to patients with dementia: Attitudes versus behaviours in nurses. *Nursing Ethics* (Nov.): 1–9.

Culley, H., Barber, R., Hope, A., & James, I. (2013). Therapeutic lying in dementia care. *Nursing Standard*, 28 (1): 35–39.

Fazio, S., Pace, D., Maslow, K., Zimmerman, S., & Kallmyer, B. (2018). Alzheimer's association dementia care practice recommendations. *Gerontologist*, 58: S1–S9.

Remington, R., Abdallah, L., Melillo, K. D., & Flanagan, J. (2006). Managing problem behaviors associated with dementia. *Rehabilitation Nursing*, 31 (5): 186–192.

Stranz, A., & Sorensdotter, R. (2016). Interpretations of person-centered dementia care: Same rhetoric, different practices? A comparative study of nursing homes in England and Sweden. *Journal of Aging Studies*, 38: 70–80.

Chapter 6: Autobiographical Memory as a Tool in Dementia Care Activities

Conway, M. A., & Pleydell-Pearce, C. W. (2000). The construction of autobiographical memories in the self-memory system. *Psychological Review*, 107 (2): 261–288.

Chapter 9: Activities of Daily Living

Maier, S., & Seligman, M. (1976). Learned helplessness: Theory and evidence. *Journal of Experimental Psychology: General*, 105 (1): 3–46.

Valkanova, V., Ebeier, K., & Allan, C. (2017). Depression is linked to dementia in older adults. *Practitioner*, 261(1800): 11–15.

Chapter 11: Lifelike Dolls and Pets

Ng, Q., Ho, C., Koh, S., Tan, W., & Chan, H. (2017). Doll therapy for dementia sufferers: A systematic review. *Complementary Therapies in Clinical Practice*, 26: 42–26.

Chapter 12: Exercise

Whitlatch, C., & Orsulic-Jeras, S. (2018). Meeting the informational, educational, and psychosocial support needs of persons living with dementia and their family caregivers. *Gerontologist*, 58 (supp. 1): S58–S73.

Chapter 13: Music

Clarke, M., Lipe, A., & Bilbrey, M. (1998). Use of music to decrease aggressive behaviours in people with dementia. *Journal of Gerontological Nursing*, 24 (7): 10–17.

Cohen, D., Post, S. G., Lo, A., Lombardo, R., & Pfeffer, B. (2018). "Music & Memory" and improved swallowing in advanced dementia. *Dementia*. https://doi.org/10.1177/1471301218769778.

Gerdner, L. A. (2000). Effects of "individualised" versus "relaxation" music on the frequency of agitation in elderly persons with Alzheimer's disease and related disorders. *International Psychogeriatrics*, 12 (1): 49–65.

Haj, M., Clement, S., Fasotti, L., & Allain, P. (2013). Effects of music on auto-biographical verbal narration in Alzheimer's disease. *Journal of Neurolinguistics*, 26 (6): 691–700.

Hall, G., & Buckwalter, K. (1987). Progressively lowered stress threshold: A conceptual model for care of adults with Alzheimer's disease. *Archives of Psychiatric Nursing*, 1 (6): 399–406.

King, J., Jones, K., Goldberg, E., Rollins, M., MacNamee, K., Moffitt, C., Naidu, S., Ferguson, M., Garcia-Leavitt, E., Amaro, J., Breitenbach, K., Watson, J., Gurgel, R., Anderson, J., & Foster, N. (2018). Increased functional connectivity after listening to favored music in adults with Alzheimer dementia. *Journal of Prevention of Alzheimer's Disease*, 19 (6): 56–62.

Koelsch, S., Gunter, T. C., Cramon, D. Y. V., Zysset, S., Lohmann, G., & Friederici, A. D. (2002). Bach speaks: A cortical "language-network" serves the processing of music. *Neuroimage*, 17 (2): 956–966.

Lin, Y., Chu, H., Yang, C., Chen, C., Chen, S., Chang, H., Hsieh, C., & Chou, K. (2011). Effectiveness of group music intervention against agitated behavior in elderly persons with dementia. *International Journal of Geriatric Psychiatry*, 26 (7): 670–678.

Lord, T. R., & Garner, J. E. (1993). Effects of music on Alzheimer patients. *Perceptual and Motor Skills*, 76 (2): 451–455.

Sherratt, K., Thornton, A., & Hatton, C. (2004). Music interventions for people with dementia: A review of the literature. *Aging and Mental Health*, 8 (1): 3–12.

Sung, H. C., Lee, W. L., Li, T. L., & Watson, R. (2012). A group music intervention using percussion instruments with familiar music to reduce anxiety and agitation of institutionalized older adults with dementia. *International Journal of Geriatric Psychiatry*, 27(6): 621–627.

Chapter 16: Hospice Activities

Chu, H., Yang, C., Lin, Y., Ou, K., Lee, T., O'Brien, A., Chou, K. (2014). The impact of group music therapy on depression and cognition in elderly persons with dementia: A randomized controlled study. *Biological Research for Nursing*, 16 (2): 209–217.

Mullen, B., Champagne, T., Krishnamurty, S., Dickson, D., & Gao, R. (2008). Exploring the safety and therapeutic effects of deep pressure stimulation using a weighted blanket. *Occupational Therapy in Mental Health*, 24 (1): 65–89.

Chapter 17: Meals and Baking

Kingston, T. (2017). Promoting fluid intake for patients with dementia or visual impairments. *British Journal of Nursing*, 26 (2): 98–99.

Chapter 18: Brain Exercise

La Rue, A. (2010). Healthy brain aging: Role of cognitive reserve, cognitive stimulation, and cognitive exercises. *Journal of Clinical Geriatric Medicine*, 26 (1): 99–111.

Chapter 19: Artwork and Creativity

Chancellor, B., Duncan, A., & Chatterjee, A. (2014). Art therapy for Alzheimer's disease and other dementias. *Journal of Alzheimer's Disease*, 39 (1): 1–11.

Mondro, A., Connell, C., Li, L., & Reed, E. (2018). Retaining identity: Creativity and caregiving. *Dementia*. https://doi.org/10.1177/1471301218803468.

Chapter 22: Sensory Rooms and Activity Boxes

Guwaldi, G. (2013). Establishing continuity of self-memory boxes in dementia facilities for older adults: Their use and usefulness. *Journal of Housing for the Elderly*, 27 (1–2): 105–119.

Hope, K. (1998). The effects of multisensory environments with older people with dementia. *Journal of Psychiatric and Mental Health Nursing*, 5 (5): 377–385.

Lorusso, L., & Bosch, S. (2018). Impact of multisensory environments on behavior for people with dementia: A systematic literature review. *Gerontologist*, 58 (3): 168–179.

Index